SAFEGUARDING
MOTHERHOOD

SAFEGUARDING MOTHERHOOD

Sol T. De Lee, M.D.

Assistant Clinical Professor of Obstetrics and Gynecology, University of Illinois; Attending Obstetrician at the Chicago Maternity Center; Former Associate in Obstetrics and Gynecology, Cook County Hospital

THIRD EDITION

With drawings by
Gladys McHugh

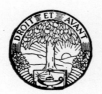

PHILADELPHIA • MONTREAL

J. B. LIPPINCOTT COMPANY

PUBLISHERS

THIS GUIDE IS DEDICATED TO MY UNCLE, DR. JOSEPH B.
DE LEE, WHO DEVOTED HIS ENTIRE BEING TO
THE WELFARE OF THE MOTHER

Foreword

Every year a large number of women and a huge number of babies lose their lives as the direct or indirect result of childbirth. Most of these deaths are preventable, and a good share of the blame for these fatalities may be attributed to the unfortunate prospective mothers themselves. Thousands of women fail to be examined by a physician during their pregnancy because of ignorance, negligence, financial difficulties, territorial inaccessibility or other reasons. These women do not call for medical assistance until they are actually ready to have their baby. Hence, they neglect to carry out specific procedures which are of the utmost importance to their own health and the welfare of the baby in their womb.

Most of the deaths from childbirth can be prevented by proper care before the baby is born and by skillful management of the actual confinement, hence every woman who is to have a baby should visit a doctor long before the expected date of confinement. In reality, a confinement case begins at the time of conception. Hence the woman should consult a physician as soon as she believes she is pregnant. The ideal arrangement is for a woman to have a thorough examination before she decides to have a baby because occasionally an abnormality is found which must be corrected in order to avoid any risk of childbirth.

The care which a woman receives before the baby arrives is known as antepartum or prenatal care. In contrast to this is the care after the child is born, and this is spoken of as postpartum or postnatal care.

In this book Doctor De Lee discusses all the important facts a pregnant woman should know about herself and her baby. These facts are so important that pregnant women who know them, and abide by them, may prevent complications which can arise during pregnancy, the actual confinement or afterwards. The illustrations drawn by Gladys McHugh are beautiful, accurate in every detail, and most instructive.

I can heartily recommend this book to prospective mothers.

J. P. Greenhill, M.D.

Preface

Having a baby should be a great adventure, for the course of pregnancy brings many new experiences. Fortunately modern science has been able to rob the adventure of nearly all its discomforts and dangers, and to bring it to a happy ending. It is necessary that the expectant mother make use of the achievements of modern medical science to provide for the well-being of both her child and herself.

The chief purposes of this small book are to inform the expectant mother regarding her pregnant condition, the means whereby her body has prepared for it, the course it will follow, and the culmination in the delivery of her child. In co-operation with her physician, it seeks to conduct her through pregnancy in a manner calculated to insure a healthy normal baby and to preserve or even improve her own mental and physical health.

The book will afford a keener insight into the "whys and wherefores" of the suggestions of her doctor. In so doing it will explain the significance of the many new sensations and reactions the pregnant woman will experience. The mention here of complications possible during pregnancy should not alarm the mother-to-be. Such complications usually can be prevented or overcome if she will follow the advice of her doctor and the simple instructions given here.

Uncommon and technical words and phrases used in the text have been explained in a glossary at the back of the book. An index of the subjects discussed has also been provided, for ease of reference.

Acknowledgments

In the composition of any book or manuscript one is dependent, at least in part, upon the writings and ideas of others. In order to present a book as all-inclusive as possible, most of the outstanding presentations written for the layman on the subject of maternal care during the past 50 years were reviewed, and many of the ideas were borrowed to serve as a basis for discussion. These works include: *Care of Mother and Child* by Clarence M. Cheadle, M.D., *Expectant Motherhood* by Nicholson J. Eastman, M.D., *What the Public Should Know About Childbirth* by Walker B. Gossett, M.D., *Approaching Motherhood* by George L. Brodhead, M.D., *The Expectant Mother* by Samuel Wyllis Bandler, M.D., *The Prospective Mother* by J. Morris Slemons, and *Modern Motherhood* by Claude Edwin Heaton, M.D. Also, the authoritative books, *The Principles and Practice of Obstetrics* by De Lee and Greenhill, and *Diseases of Children* by Holt and McIntosh were used as references.

In addition to these sources of information, I had the privilege of having the personal interest and aid of Dr. Edith Potter, a specialist in the pathology of the newborn at the Chicago Lying-in Hospital; Dr. A. J. Halpern, author of the widely accepted book, *How to Raise a Healthy Baby;* Miss Anne Kirchner, Superintendent of Nurses at the Chicago Lying-in Hospital; and Mesdames M. T. Straube and K. Grosnickel, dieticians at the same institution.

Miss Ethel W. Ransom, R.N., Chief of the Nursing of the Baby Development Clinic of Chicago, edited the Baby's Needs portion of the chapter, The Newborn.

I am also indebted to several friends for their helpful criticism, including Jane Hess, Betty Bergman, Elaine Glazer and Jeanne Gross. Iva Duncan's suggestions and co-operation have consistently been most valuable.

The drawings which appear in this book were made by Gladys McHugh, a noted medical artist. She has drawn many illustrations for standard textbooks, including those of Dr. J. B. De Lee, Dr. F. L. Adair, and others. Also she has several works of her own on the complicated anatomy of the eye and the ear which have received wide recognition.

Contents

1

Introduction

Guarded by modern medical science, childbirth is no longer a miracle but a safe and satisfying, if somewhat tedious, experience.

Upon you who have conceived a new life there rests a great responsibility—a responsibility which, if accepted seriously and carried out intelligently, brings reward beyond compare. To your child you owe a sound development; to yourself you owe a trouble-free pregnancy. The achievement of each of these depends upon you. Your reward is the untold happiness derived from a sturdy, healthy baby and a future free from those conditions that are the result of mismanaged childbirth.

There still remain today too many persons who suffer under the delusion that once conception has occurred, all that the child will be at birth is already determined, and hence that whatever happens during pregnancy is unimportant to the well-being of the unborn. This idea is not justified. Conception sets only the upper limit on the qualities the child may attain if he grows under ideal conditions within the mother. It is up to you, who are carrying a child, to see that your baby receives the maximum of his inheritance by seeking the skilled medical guidance that will keep your health at its highest level. Adopt a safe and sane attitude toward your condition. Nine months slip by quickly if you check any tendency toward emotional upset. Not only your child but you yourself will benefit if the doctor does not have to counteract the effects of poor diet, overwork, emotional strain, and careless actions. Antepartum, or prenatal care, should be sought early after conception has taken place because medical supervision is the best insurance for a sound baby, safe delivery, and the healthy future of the mother.

The purpose of prenatal care is to avoid, arrest, or cure disorders and deficiencies which may prove injurious to the mother, the unborn child or to both. It brings the woman to labor in a physical condition adequate to withstand the unavoidable strain and assures her of a successful delivery and a prompt recovery. The value of prenatal guidance is similar to that of periodic health examinations since both stress intelligent supervision, prevention or early discovery of illness, proper treatment and follow-up of each case. Such care is absolutely necessary for some women if they are to avoid calamity; it is helpful to all. There is no other field in preventive medicine that offers such remarkable returns in sparing human life and suffering.

A quarter of a century ago prenatal care was almost unheard of. It was customary for the patient or her family to see a doctor once during her pregnancy and then merely to arrange for him to attend the confinement. Only the occurrence of unusual and possibly ominous symptoms brought the patient to call her doctor before labor began. Little importance was attached to diet though now physicians are aware that the proper diet prevents many difficulties then common during pregnancy. Patients rarely were weighed with any regularity—the weight gain was held to be unimportant. The blood pressure and urine were almost completely ignored, though now the doctor examines both frequently. The existence of syphilis often escaped attention and as a result both mother and baby suffered. Conditions often existed which did not impair the general health of the patient and yet presented obstetrical difficulties. Because of the former prevalence of bone deformities due to rickets, contracted pelves were more common several decades ago than they are now. Such pelves were the basis of difficult and often unsuccessful labors which not infrequently terminated in the invalidism or death of mother and baby. Patients were allowed to go into labor without being checked as to pelvic size and type. Such information is now obtained routinely and an unusual condition is rarely a hazard.

While pregnancy is a normal physiologic process, not all women who become pregnant are normal physiologically. For example, a woman's kidneys may have been impaired by scarlet fever or other infection and yet exhibit no sign of weakness until the strain of pregnancy is thrown upon them. Tuberculosis is common, and if present, increases temporarily or permanently the hazard of childbearing. Cardiac disease is relatively common and handicaps the prospective mother, especially during labor. Problems such as these should be recognized early in, if not prior to, pregnancy.

The early diagnosis of constitutional diseases coincident with pregnancy is not the only advantage of prenatal care. So too is the discovery of those conditions which result directly from the pregnancy itself. For a little-understood reason, some patients develop a poisoning or toxemia of pregnancy which, in the form of eclampsia can be very serious in its effects on both the mother and baby. In recent years fewer and fewer prospective mothers have suffered from this condition. The explanation is quite obvious: prenatal care alone explains why this number has diminished and is still decreasing. Patients are being educated to seek factor such as an underactive thyroid gland, which the doctor will discover.

THE PHYSICAL EXAMINATION— THE SIGNS

The signs of pregnancy are those changes which can be objectively observed by the patient or doctor or both. Early in pregnancy the signs can be confused with other conditions and therefore, are called "presumptive" if occasionally found in pregnancy, "probable" if usually found, whereas starting with the last half of pregnancy there can be little doubt about the patient's condition and the characteristic signs are called "positive."

Probable Signs

Changes in the Skin. Starting from the beginning of pregnancy, certain areas of the skin gradually become more heavily pigmented. Pigmentation, localized at first about the nipples and in a straight line down the middle of the abdomen, may become quite evident about the end of the second month. In the form of blotches, pigmentation may appear about the face, hands, or any part of the body. This condition is sometimes referred to as the "mask of pregnancy" when the face is involved, or as "liver spots" when present on other parts of the body. The latter is an unfortunate name, implying as it does a disorder of the liver, which is in no way involved. The condition is, in all events, only temporary, and disappears after childbirth.

Another condition of the skin found in some pregnancies is known as striae. Striae are pinkish lines observed about the abdomen, breasts, thighs. They sometimes produce a feeling of itchiness and a sensation of superficial tenderness. After pregnancy these striae become white and nearly unnoticeable.

More rare than the foregoing symptoms is the occasional appearance over the surface of the body, and especially on the face, of fine hair. It almost invariably disappears soon after the baby is born.

Breast Changes. The changing condition of the breasts during pregnancy has been described in the preceding section.

Vaginal Changes. Very early in pregnancy the lining of the vagina becomes darkened, the tip of the womb softens, and the womb itself becomes enlarged and softened. Considering these changes in combination with the other symptoms of the patient, the physician can state, not positively, but with a fair degree of certainty, whether or not the patient is pregnant.

Increase in Size of Abdomen. At about three and one half or four months, in the patient of average size, there is a slight bulge of the lower abdomen due to the growth of the womb. Its presence is, therefore, only probable evidence of pregnancy because a similar contour may be caused by a tumor.

Positive Signs

Fetal Outline and Movements. At approximately the fifth month the doctor can detect, either by touch or by direct vision, movements of the baby, and can outline, by palpating the abdomen, the fetal parts. This is positive evidence of pregnancy.

Fetal Heart Beat. At around four and one half months the doctor is able to listen through a stethoscope and hear the baby's heart beat. It sounds to him like a watch ticking at a distance. The rate of the heart differs from that of the mother's, being approximately 160 beats per minute early in pregnancy and a little slower later. This is positive evidence in itself of pregnancy.

X-Ray. Occasionally a doctor will be in doubt about the patient's condition even as late as the fourth or fifth month, at which time it is possible to visualize the fetal skeleton by x-ray. At that time, or at any time thereafter, the question of a multiple pregnancy can be answered.

Laboratory Tests. We are indebted to Aschheim and Zondek for the discoveries which form the basis of our most reliable laboratory tests for pregnancy. The tests are just short of 100 per cent accurate, and when the results are considered together with the other conditions present, the doctor can be quite certain of the diagnosis.

The tests are performed by injecting either the blood or the urine of a possibly pregnant woman into a rabbit, rat or mouse. Even a particular species of frog has been used for such biologic assay. The tests are reliable even when made very soon

after conception; a high degree of accuracy has been obtained for almost any time after two weeks beyond the missed menstrual period.

Now that the patient has confirmed the existence of her pregnancy she will be actively concerned in safeguarding herself and her child, and in assisting the doctor's efforts to insure that both will go through to delivery in good condition. It is only logical that certain problems enter the prospective mother's mind and such questions as "When will my baby arrive?," "What hospital will I go to?," "How much is this going to cost?," and "How often do I see the doctor?," have to be given consideration. It is therefore timely to discuss these and related questions.

REPEAT VISITS TO THE DOCTOR

The patient is seen each third week during the first seven months and every second week about the eighth month and once every week during the last month—more often if deemed advisable. She should bring with her each time a three-ounce (3 oz.) specimen of urine in a clean bottle on which is written her name.

On these subsequent visits the patient's condition will be discussed and questions will be answered. It is an excellent idea for the patient to write down her questions, for these often escape her memory at the appointed time, only to return after the patient has finished her visit. In the back of the book, on page 119, will be found a convenient place to record the patient's questions and the doctor's suggestions. Also at these visits, the patient will have the examinations that are necessary. Abdominal, vaginal and laboratory examinations will be done as indicated. She can expect to be weighed and have her blood pressure taken each time, and to be questioned for the presence of unusual symptoms.

DATE OF CONFINEMENT

It is impossible to predict accurately the day when a baby is to arrive. However, the approximate date can be determined in a number of ways.

1. Add seven days to the first day of the last monthly flow and subtract three months. Thus, if the last menstrual period began July 10, add seven days, giving July 17, and subtract three months, which gives April 17 as the approximate day labor may be expected. In most cases confinement will take place within a few days before or after this calculated date.

2. A woman having her first baby may add 22 weeks to the day she first feels the baby move, these first movements being known as "quickening." A woman who has already borne children should add 24 weeks.

3. If the exact day of conception is known, 273 days added to this will give the approximate date of confinement. (Conception takes place almost invariably on or about 14 days previous to a menstrual period, regardless of the length of the menstrual cycle; a small percentage of women ovulate at a time not consistent with this pattern.)

4. By repeated examinations, a physician can usually tell approximately when a baby will be born. This is based upon the fact that during pregnancy the womb enlarges at a constant rate. Such alterations in the level of the top of the uterus in relation to the navel and lower rib margin indicate quite satisfactorily the month to which pregnancy has advanced and will aid in making a prediction as to the date of confinement.

PROLONGED PREGNANCY

As you know, especially after reading the above, the actual date of confinement is just as likely to be a few days before as after the expected day given. Patients usually express joy in having a baby delivered a little before term. But the period beyond this time is a most trying and irksome one. Each day seems longer than the one before, and the patient's emotional condition and that of her immediate family often become upset. Because of this, mothers frequently request that something be done to start labor. As a rule this is an unwise procedure, and most doctors will not be influenced merely by the patient's wishes in the matter. Such arbitrary inductions of labor are not without complications, and it is only in the presence of a real indication, or where the doctor feels that the baby is postmature, that steps will be taken to cause labor to begin. There is an old saying that "when the fruit is ripe it will fall from the tree." This analogy is quite appropriate and should not be forgotten by the anxious expectant mother.

If the doctor feels, on the basis of the history and his repeated examinations, that he is dealing with a case of true postmaturity, labor will be induced. The exact manner varies with the doctor in charge and may include the use of castor oil, an enema, quinine, pituitrin, or rupturing the bag of waters.

The actual reasons for an apparent prolonged pregnancy are:

1. A miscalculation on the part of the patient; that is, she has forgotten the actual date of her last menstrual period.

2. The patient may get pregnant 20 days or so after her last menstrual period instead of at the mid-menstrual time, thus making the date of confinement seven to ten days beyond that calculated by our usual method.

3. Pregnancies are a bit longer in patients who have long menstrual cycles (35 days) than in those who have short menstrual cycles (25 days).

Hospital Reservation

A hospital room will be reserved for the patient at the first prenatal visit. Because of the uncertainty of the date of labor, the hospital management cannot promise to have any particular room available, but it will do all it can to meet the patient's needs and desires.

Hospital Rules

The rules prescribed by the hospital should be obeyed. Relatives and friends should be urged to observe the regulations carefully. Never forget that these rules and regulations, though sometimes apparently too strict, are the result of years of experience and of intense study of conditions and are first, last and always intended to promote the welfare of the mothers and their babies.

Children are not allowed to visit in a hospital for they sometimes carry the scarlet fever or diphtheria germ. No visitor should enter the hospital who has been near a person who has a contagious disease or has recently recovered from one herself.

The Fee

The hospital charges according to the type of accommodations the patient receives. Private rooms are more expensive than the semiprivate, as would be expected, but otherwise the hospital charges (delivery room, anesthetic, etc.) are the same. The doctor's fee includes routine visits, a normal delivery, hospital care and routine attention to six weeks after delivery. Arrangements should be made during an early visit as to the manner of caring for this.

Articles to Take to the Hospital

A patient who belongs to the Blue Cross or other hospital service plan should take her identification card with her to the hospital.

The mother should pack her bag some day well in advance of the expected day of confinement, as a matter of expediency. The articles suggested are not absolutely essential but will make the hospital stay more comfortable and pleasant.

Gowns (These are furnished but are very plain. Most patients prefer their own after a few days)
Bed jacket
Dressing robe
Bedroom slippers
Brassiere, regular
Brassiere, nursing (2)
Sanitary belt (pads are furnished by hospital)
Underwear
Comb, brush and hand-mirror
Toothbrush and paste
Talcum powder
Cologne or toilet water
Cosmetics
Manicure set
Clock or watch
Fountain pen, stationery and stamps
A book or two

Most hospitals provide all that is necessary for the baby during its stay, but an outfit for going home is required. This can be taken to the hospital along with the mother's things or brought later by the husband.

HOME DELIVERY

Today fewer women are being delivered of their babies at home. This is accounted for by the popularization of hospitals because of their greater conveniences for mothers and doctors, improved incomes and hospitalization insurance, and the chance for a rest for those mothers who have other children at home is also an inducement. Also, women feel safer delivering in a hospital. Generally speaking, if an ideal technic has not been worked out, this is a well founded feeling—certainly for complicated cases. On the other hand, most cases are normal and such cases can be safely conducted at home with the proper medical supplies and assistance. The woman who desires to have a home confinement should so inform her doctor. He can then instruct her what paraphernalia to have in readiness and make the necessary arrangements.

3

The Anatomy and Physiology of Reproduction

Whoever considers the study of anatomy will never be an atheist. I hold it to be the greatest miracle in nature.
LORD HERBERT

The body undergoes from infancy changes which prepare the adult to reproduce. In order to understand the adjustments which take place within her during pregnancy, the patient should know something about the skeleton, the generative organs and the physiologic developments which are brought to a climax in the delivery of the mature infant.

ANATOMY

The female reproductive system is comprised of the external generative organs, the internal generative organs and the breasts. Although the pelvis is not included in this system, it may influence the birth process and so it will be briefly discussed.

Pelvis. The strong hollow bony support by which the lower extremities are attached to the trunk is the pelvis. Its upper portion, which is not important insofar as childbearing is concerned, is known as the false pelvis; the lower portion is the smaller true pelvis, the bony part of the birth canal itself. Within the

pelvic region are the organs of reproduction. Most women have a pelvis well suited for childbearing, a so-called normal pelvis. It is possible that, due to heredity, disease or accident, a pelvis may be abnormally contracted, making natural delivery or any delivery from the vagina an impossibility. Prenatal care will at once reveal any gross abnormality. In the borderline cases where there is reasonable doubt about the adequacy of the pelvis, the vigilance of the physician will eliminate any danger from an unsuspected disproportion between the baby's head and the pelvis.

External Generative Organs. Those structures which are visible on inspection are called the vulva. The vulva consists of two pairs of labia or lips, and within them are the clitoris, the vestibule, the hymen and the introitus or entrance to the vagina. The outer large labia or labia majora join above the introitus in a pad of fat over the pubic bone. Below and behind they meet at a point known as the perineum —a wide muscular structure important in the support of the pelvic floor. It separates the genitalia from the anus or opening of the lower bowel. Within the large labia lie the labia minora which enclose an tubes and ovaries. Because of their complex structure and importance they shall be described individually.

The vagina is a muscular, highly dilatable canal lined by mucous membrane. From its attachment to the cervix (the neck of the uterus)

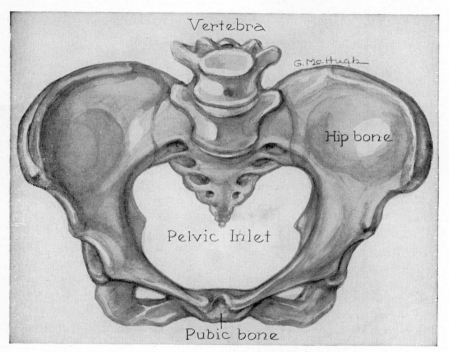

Vertebra

G. McHugh

Hip bone

Pelvic Inlet

Pubic bone

FIG. 2. Normal female pelvis.

almond-shaped opening known as the vestibule. They meet above the vestibule at the site of the clitoris, a sensitive erectile structure important in its relation to sexual stimulations. The introitus is directed inward from the vestibule and is surrounded wholly by the hymen.

Internal Generative Organs. These include the vagina, uterus, above, it extends to the vestibule of the external genitalia below, where it opens to the exterior. Its orifice is partially covered or enclosed by a fold of connective tissue called the hymen. The vagina is the organ of copulation and acts as a receptacle for the male semen.

The uterus, or womb, is an unpaired muscular organ situated in

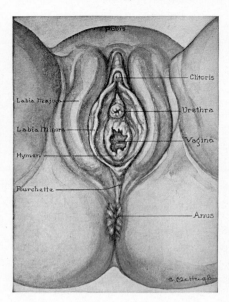

Labia Majora

Labia Minora

Hymen

Fourchette

Clitoris

Urethra

Vagina

Anus

C. McHugh

FIG. 3. External genitalia viewed
from below.

the true pelvis, supported by the
pelvic floor and various ligaments.
It lies between the bladder in front
and the rectum behind. It is divided
into two portions, the cervix or neck,
and the corpus or body. The former
lies in the vagina, the latter above it.
The uterus is extremely important in
several respects. It is the organ
directly associated with the menstrual cycle, a process which prepares
the womb for the fertilized ovum.
During pregnancy it receives the
fertilized egg and is the site of its
growth and development. Finally, it
is an expulsive organ, enabling the
baby to be born by the efforts of its
muscular contractions. At this time,
when the ovum has developed into
a baby, the cervix is no longer a

narrow canal but, possessing the
quality of great dilation, becomes a
wide, open passageway. (See Chapter 9, The Labor.)

The fallopian tubes are also
known as oviducts for they serve
to convey the ova, or eggs, to the
uterus. They are paired tubular
structures, about five inches in
length, each forming a continuation
of the two upper, outer portions of
the uterus. They are continuous with
the uterus and run laterally to lie at
their outer ends adjacent to the
ovaries.

The tubes are muscular and undergo rhythmic contractions, a factor
not only in the transportation of the
fertilized ovum down their length
to the uterine cavity but probably
important in receiving the ovum
from the ovary by way of their
trumpet-shaped openings.

The ovaries are the female sex
glands. They are paired organs situated one on either side of the uterus,
immediately adjacent to it, and located just below the fallopian tubes.
Each is about the size and shape of
an unshelled almond.

The ovaries are extremely important structures. They are the source
of hormones which affect not only
the ovaries themselves, but the entire
body and its functions. The development of the sexual structure into
functioning and useful organs and
the appearance of the sexual characteristics in puberty are all the result
of the action of the ovarian hormones. The ovaries function under
the influence of the pituitary gland,

the so-called "motor of the ovary." Furthermore, the ovaries contain many thousands of ova, one of which during each menstrual cycle reaches maturity and is expelled. This is the process known as ovulation.

15 to 24 lobes, each of which is a secreting gland subdivided into several lobules. Each lobule has a small duct or passageway which unites with others to form a large duct for each lobe, each large duct having a

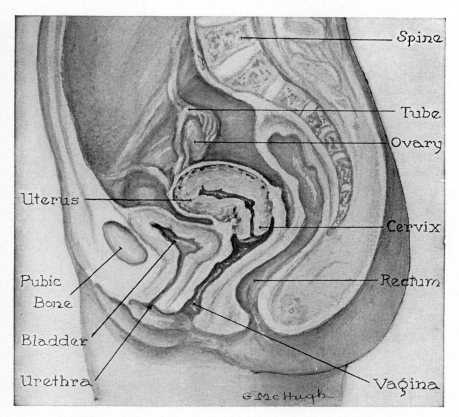

FIG. 4. Midline section through the pelvis viewed from the side, showing relationship of uterus to the bladder and rectum.

The breasts are modified skin glands and are also known as mammary glands. They begin to enlarge at puberty and during pregnancy undergo further growth and development. Each breast is divided into

minute opening at the nipple. The lobules contain many small irregular pouches called acini which secrete milk into the smallest of the ducts.

Surrounding the nipple is a pigmented area called the areola in

which there are many small eleva-
tions known as Montgomery's
glands or tubercles. The enlargement
of these is of no particular significance, merely one of the changes
noted during pregnancy.

The female breasts are capable of

infant food, and the way the infant
should be put to the breast are all
discussed in Chapter 10, Convalescence and After-Care.

PHYSIOLOGY

Puberty is the period when the

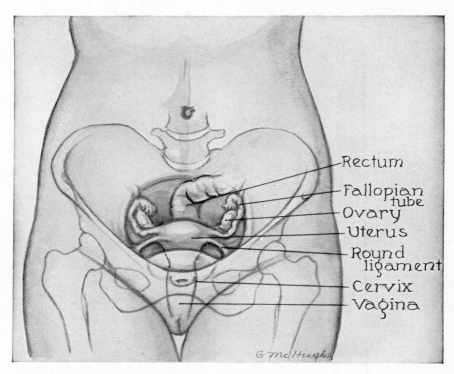

FIG. 5. Structures of the female as they lie in the pelvis which is shown in
outline—front view.

amazing production. The size and
shape do not indicate their ability to
secrete milk. Many other factors,
especially the mental attitude, are
influential in this function. The factors influencing the quantity and
quality of breast milk, the superiority
of breast milk over all other types of

individual first becomes capable of
reproduction. This occurs in girls
at an average age of 13, with a
normal range of from 11 to 16 years.
This phase of development involves
a series of physical and mental alterations, and is indicated by the appearance of the secondary sexual

characteristics. The physical changes include menstruation, breast growth, widening of the hips, female distribution of hair, and changes in the voice. Mentally, there is an awareness of these bodily changes and an increased consciousness of sex.

The basis for this development lies in the changing activities of the endocrine or ductless gland system,

Puberty is a critical phase in a child's life and particularly a girl's unless she is informed and prepared for it. Undesirable and far-reaching emotional reactions can develop. These emotions are largely prevented by a matter-of-fact, intelligent educational program conducted by the parents or teachers to advise the child of the physical and social character-

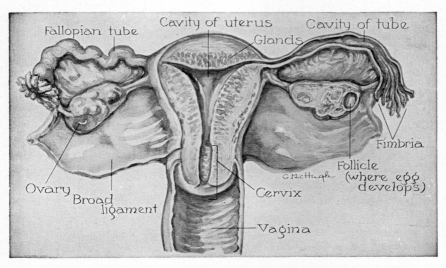

FIG. 6. The organs of reproduction viewed from behind with the uterus, right tube and ovary in cross-section.

which manufactures products called hormones that are secreted directly into the blood stream as it flows through the substance of the glands. In relation to the generative system, the most important of the ductless glands are the pituitary, the ovaries and the thyroid, all intimately related and secreting hormones which affect the function of each other, the body generally, and usually themselves.

istics of her growth and development.

The Menstrual Cycle. Ordinarily childbearing is possible only from the time of puberty until the menopause; that is, from the onset of menstruation to its cessation. Of course, there are many exceptions on record, the extremes being medical curiosities. The menstrual cycle plays a vital role in childbearing. Only rarely can conception take place where menstruation does not occur. This is partly because ovulation rarely occurs without rhythmic bleeding and because menstruation is associated with preparatory changes

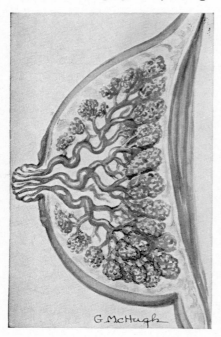

Fig. 7. A schematic drawing of the milk-forming structures of the breast during pregnancy. Clusters of tiny sacs (acini) produce the milk which is carried through tubules to the nipple.

in the uterus which make it suitable to become the fertilized ovum's final destination.

During the menstrual cycle, usually 28 days in length but often normal even when 21 or 35 days, there are numerous physiologic changes taking place in many organs of the body, especially those directly concerned with reproduction—the uterus and the ovaries. The organ of menstruation, the uterus, shows marked fluctuations in the character of its lining. Immediately after menstruation this is very thin, just a fine layer. Gradually this lining increases in thickness until a week before the next menstruation is expected. Then it is many layers in depth, soft and velvety, infiltrated with myriads of small vessels which give it a rich blood supply and a soft, spongy texture. It is here the ovum implants itself if it has been fertilized. If fertilization has not occurred, this uterine lining soon disintegrates and becomes a mixture of tissue and blood which flows from the uterine cavity to the outside. The menstrual flow carries in its stream the unfertilized ovum. Normally, the menstrual flow lasts from three to seven days.

Menopause. The termination of the woman's menstrual career is known as the menopause. It is the cessation of not only menstruation but almost invariably of ovulation as well. Sometimes a woman who is at or near the menopause interprets the cessation of flow as the beginning of that event, only to find that she has actually conceived. Individuals have been known to become pregnant even years after the menopause, indicating that, while uncommon, ovulation can occur without menstruation. Children so conceived are often referred to by the laity as "change-of-life babies."

In most women, the menopause

occurs somewhere between the ages of 42 and 48 and is frequently attended by symptoms which are characteristic of this phase—hot flashes, irritability, headaches and emotional instability. With the proper medical guidance most, if not all, of the discomforts of this phase of a woman's life can be alleviated.

Ovulation. It was mentioned that the ovary contains many thousands of ova. The ovum that is going to be capable of fertilization undergoes a series of changes before it reaches maturity. When it finally does mature, it lies in a fluid cavity toward the surface of the ovary known as a graafian follicle. The rupture of this sac and simultaneous expulsion of the egg are known as ovulation. This occurs approximately 14 days before the next anticipated menstrual period, regardless of the length of the cycle, or at the midmenstrual period in a 28-day cycle. Some women feel a slight pain over one ovary at this time, others notice a small spot of blood, and most women have a slight rise in their body temperature. This rise in the body temperature is important in sterility cases, for it is a definite advantage to know when a woman is most fertile. This is also of benefit to those who seek contraceptive advice, for the days distant from this time of temperature rise are infertile ones. The "safe period" is the time when a woman is not fertile and is usually one week after and one week before menstruation, but ovulation at times fails to follow a definite pattern and conception is known to have occurred at any time during the menstrual cycle.

When ovulation occurs, the cavity of the follicle undergoes certain changes with the formation of a yellowish structure known as a corpus luteum. When fertilization has taken place this is called a corpus luteum of pregnancy. It is a temporary gland of internal secretion and produces a hormone called progesterone, important to the maintenance of the pregnancy. Lack of the hormone has been blamed for many spontaneous abortions and is given consideration in their prevention.

What happens to this ovum which has escaped from the follicle? It passes into the nearer fallopian tube in a little-understood manner and is carried down the tube toward the uterus. During this trip the ovum may meet a sperm and be fertilized or it may pass into the uterus unfertilized and be removed with the next menstrual flow.

FETAL DEVELOPMENT AND GROWTH

An explanation of the development of any living organism should begin with a description of its fundamental unit of structure—the cell. The structural basis of all parts of the human body is the cell. All the cells throughout the body are fundamentally similar in structure and function. However, their appearance varies as they become specialized to perform one predominant function such as secretion by gland cells or contraction by muscle cells. Combined they form tissues of many diverse shapes and purposes. Each cell is a minute portion of living matter or protoplasm separated from the other cells by an envelope, the cell membrane. Each cell has its own center of activity, the nucleus. Cells are arranged into groups to form tissues and organs, as the heart, kidney or skin. The manner of their organization and the specialized nature of the cells determine the function the organ or tissue can and will perform.

Germinal Cells. The female germinal or reproductive cell is an ovum. It has been estimated that each ovary contains about 20,000 ova at birth, though not a single one ripens until the time of puberty. From puberty to the menopause, the duration of the menstruating period, one ovum ripens each month. Rarely more than one ovum ripens and this makes possible the occurrence of one type of multiple birth.

The human ovum is a minute structure measuring about 1/125 of an inch in diameter, and is hardly visible to the naked eye. It is a single cell containing a nucleus and its surrounding nutritive material, the yolk.

Once the ovum ripens it is magically transported to the oviduct, having been expelled by rupture of its follicle, its home in the ovary. The life of the egg is a matter of hours and just how many is as yet not known. Some investigations have shown it to be as high as 18 and others as few as 8. In the tube the fate of the ovum is decided; it either passes unchanged into the uterus or is stimulated to a remarkable metamorphosis by contact with the male germinal cell. The latter cell is like the ovum in its possession of a nucleus but otherwise appears quite different. Their sizes relative to one another can be seen in the illustration. The sperm consists of a head containing the nucleus and a tail which enables it to travel under its own power. It must travel upward to the outer end of the tube where it meets the ovum. Nature has increased the likelihood that there will be a partner for the ovum by providing hundreds of millions of these motile bodies in each ejaculation of a normal healthy male. Although millions of them die in the vagina as a result of the acid secretion there, myriads survive to travel up through the cervix and uterus to the tubes where they attempt to invade the ovum. In addition to being produced in vastly greater numbers than the female germinal cells, the sperm are also more hardy. They have been known to survive for as long as two or three days within the fallopian tube.

Fertilization. The ovum attracts the sperm almost as a magnet does iron filings. When the two types of germinal cells lie in the oviducts, the spermatozoa seethe around the ovum and one (just one) penetrates it. The moment they touch, the two cells unite so intimately that all traces of the spermatozoon are lost. This process, known as fertilization, has as its main purpose the union of the two nuclei of the male and female germinal cell. The laity rightly speak of fertilization as conception, for at this instant a new individual begins his existence.

Physical and mental potentialities, sex and the other hereditary traits are all determined from the moment of fertilization. The sperm constitutes the total contribution of the male parent to pregnancy and to the inherited traits of his child; the ovum, the entire female contribution. Thus to attain full development the fertilized ovum now needs only a place to grow and a source of nourishment.

First Steps in Development— Cell Division. The dawn of development in the fertilized ovum is signaled by unusual activity within the cell followed by alterations upon its surface. As the ovum lies in the tube, its surface indents and the cell divides to form two cells in place of one. These cells in turn divide, yielding four which grow and divide into eight. In this manner the single cell rapidly becomes a multitude of cells clinging together in the shape of a sphere, which is solid at first but soon becomes hollow like a mulberry.

While these changes are occurring the fertilized ovum is transported a distance of four to six inches down the tube and comes to rest in the uterus, where it will complete its development. The journey requires about seven days and is made possible by rhythmic contractions of the tube, and by a downward current created by the wavelike action of myriads of fine hairy structures protruding into its interior.

Implantation. As the fertilized ovum is undergoing these changes and making its journey, the womb is completing preparations to receive it. By the time the new boarder has become capable of attaching itself to the wall of the uterus for its lengthy stay, the latter has attained its optimum condition for this event. The lining has reached its greatest thickness and succulence; it is soft and vascular with a countless number of tiny blood vessels distributed throughout its width and depth. Upon reaching the uterus, the ovum merely rests there for about one week, while it undergoes further alterations in structure so that it may successfully embed itself in the uterine wall.

To further its purpose of obtaining nourishment for the ovum and to eliminate waste products, the outer layer soon sends out villi, which are finger-like projections that dip like the roots of a tree into these blood-filled spaces. The villi themselves contain microscopic blood vessels which carry from the surrounding blood the nutritive materials necessary for growth and development and carry to it the products of metabolism, the waste materials.

The fertilized ovum is able to embed itself in the wall of the uterus only because of the action of this outer layer of cells, the trophoblast. These outer cells digest tissue with which they come in contact, not only accomplishing the above, but they also perforate the many small blood vessels lying within the uterine wall, laying open the mother's blood stream in a definite organized fashion. The ovum thus finds itself sunk in the soft tissue of the uterus with tiny pools of blood everywhere as a ball of cells, having the appearance of a mulberry though very much smaller. At one point inside this little sac a new cluster of cells appears and hangs toward the center. This is known as the internal cell mass and it is of greatest importance for it is from these cells alone that

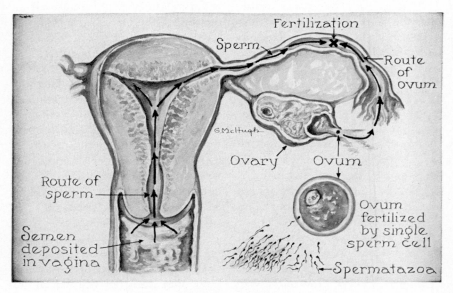

Fig. 8. The process of fertilization. Note the ovum leaving the ovarian follicle and its subsequent course into the tube. Sperm deposited in the vagina travel upward through the cervix and uterus into the outer end of the tube where fertilization takes place. The insert shows the relative sizes of the sperm and ovum.

around it. Thus one can see that the blood of the mother is separated from that of the embryo, for the cell walls of the villi intervene. The villi which penetrate the uterine wall plus the wall itself at that point form an organ called the placenta.

Embryo, Placenta, Umbilical Cord and Bag of Waters. We left the ovum a few paragraphs ago the baby develops. The duty of the other outer cells or trophoblastic layer was just described above.

From now on the cells which compose the entire mass rapidly increase in number and become more diverse in character. These different kinds of cells rearrange themselves and multiply and some of them begin to form the different parts of the baby's body while others develop into two thin membranes that finally enclose the embryo in a double sac. The embryo stage lasts five weeks, during which time the structure of the individual appears and the pattern of the organs is arranged. Thus the "bag of waters," but doctors refer to it as the membranes. As it enlarges and pushes out into the uterine cavity it still consists of two thin membranes except where it is attached to the uterus, at which point it grows into a thick, spongy mass

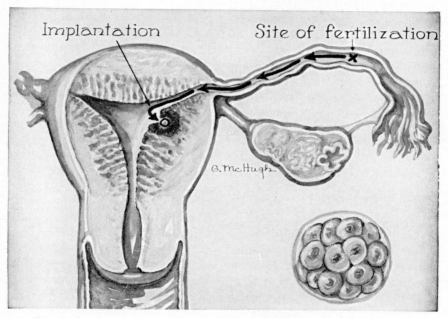

Implantation   Site of fertilization

FIG. 9. Implantation. Following fertilization the ovum subdivides into a cluster of cells as it descends into the uterus, where it burrows into the thick lining. Insert: The group of cells (magnified) into which the fertilized ovum has divided by the time implantation takes place.

at an amazingly early period the baby's structure has been defined. The embryo is now attached to the inner surface of the sac; the space which it does not occupy is filled with fluid and the sac itself is attached to the uterine lining at the point where the cell mass happened to stop and bury itself.

This sac is what is popularly called of projections, the villi, containing the fetal blood vessels as described. Doctors refer to the villi and that part of the lining of the womb into which they sink as the placenta. It is also called the "afterbirth" because it is expelled after the baby is born. When fully developed at two months the placenta is a round disklike structure. At full term the placenta is a fleshy organ measuring about eight inches in diameter and one inch in thickness.

As the baby's development advances, the part by which he is connected with the placenta at the navel lengthens into what is called the umbilical cord. At full term this is about 20 inches long and one half inch in diameter. In this cord are blood vessels which lie close together and are encased in a heavy jellylike substance that protects them from injury. Through these vessels blood constantly flows back and forth, carrying nourishment to the baby from the mother and waste matter from the little body to the placenta where it is taken up by her blood.

Month-by-Month Development of the Baby

The passage of each lunar month after conception brings a marked change in the stage of development the baby has reached. It must be recalled that conception occurs usually two weeks after the last menstrual period and that the baby is not a month old until two weeks after the first missed menstrual period. The age of the baby is given in terms of lunar months or four-week periods; this is a convenient basis of calculation, for such a month corresponds to the usual length of the menstrual cycle.

End of First Lunar Month. The sac is the size of a pigeon's egg, the outer surface of which is lined with a membrane, called the chorion, covered with villi. The umbilical cord is not yet formed. A mouth and jaw are present although the eyes, ears and nose are not apparent. The backbone has been formed and is greatly bent on itself, so much so that the head is near the tip of the tail (a tail which is soon to disappear). A rudimentary heart has been formed and pulsates regularly, sending blood along the tiny vessels which are distributed throughout the embryo.

The beginnings of the future digestive system are visible—a long slender tube leading from the mouth to a bulge in this tube, the eventual stomach, running from which are the rudimentary intestines. Small budlike projections represent the sites of future arms and legs.

End of Second Lunar Month. The embryo is one inch long and is bent on itself. From this point on till birth the embryo is referred to as a "fetus." The fetus now has a head which has grown quite large, due to the development of the brain. The nubbins at the site of the extremities grow in length and each divides into three parts—the arms, forearms and hands, the thighs, legs and feet; the hands and feet are webbed. The tail is being absorbed. The external genitalia appear, but sex is not distinguishable.

End of Third Lunar Month. The fetus begins to look more like a baby. It has increased its length threefold in the past month, and weighs an ounce. Sex can be distinguished. Movements begin at this time but are too slight to be felt by the mother. The umbilical cord is forming.

End of Fourth Lunar Month. The fetus is now six and one half inches long and weighs about four ounces. The baby's body is covered with fine hair, called lanugo. The placenta and umbilical cord are well formed. Fetal movements are

End of Sixth Lunar Month. The baby is now one foot long and weighs one and one half pounds. The skin is wrinkled and red and the head is still large in proportion to the body. The eyebrows and lashes are formed and the eyelids separated. If born, the fetus may live and move its limbs freely for a short time

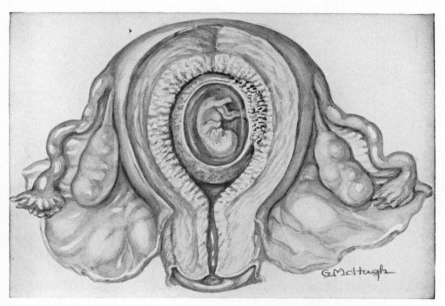

Fig. 10. Two-month embryo implanted in the uterus—life size.

stronger but usually not felt by the mother, though some multiparas will note them.

End of Fifth Lunar Month. The length of the fetus is about ten inches and it weighs one half pound. Quickening is definitely experienced and the doctor is able to hear the fetal heart beat. Lanugo hair is still present and a small amount of typical hair is on the head.

but dies since the respiratory organs are not developed.

End of Seventh Lunar Month. The fetus now measures about 15 inches and weighs approximately two and one half pounds. The baby looks like a thin wrinkled little old man and has a very weak cry. If born at this time its chances of survival are about one in ten though they may be bettered under ideal conditions.

End of Eighth Lunar Month.
The fetus measures about 16 inches
and weighs four pounds. With good
nursing care, babies born at this stage
have a much better than even chance
mature infant, though if born its
chances of survival are not quite as
good as if delivered four weeks later,
or full term. It has a length of about
a foot and a half and weighs ap-

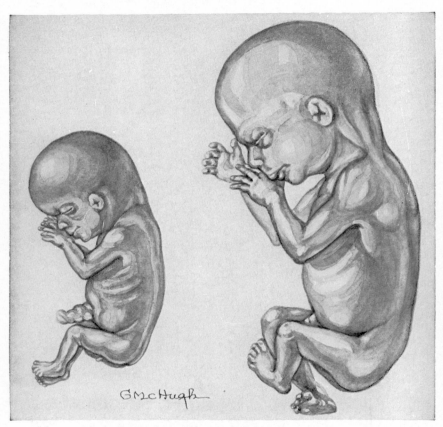

FIG. 11. (*Left*) Three-month fetus. (*Right*) Four-month fetus.
Both drawn actual size.

of survival, certainly better than if
born as a seven-month baby. (See
Chapter 4, Mental Attitude and
Beliefs.)
End of the Ninth Lunar Month.
The fetus can now be considered a
proximately six pounds, and but for
a more mature appearance due to the
increase in length and weight (it
gains about one-half pound a week
during the last two months) it
changes very little from now on.

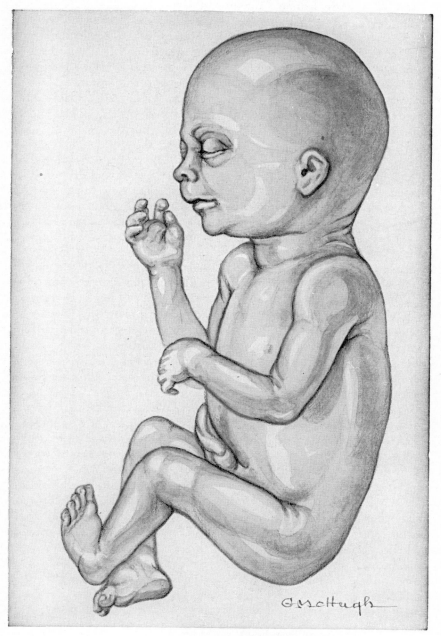

F<small>IG</small>. 12. Five-month fetus—actual size.

End of Tenth Lunar Month.
The fetus is at full term with a usual
length of about 20 inches and weighs
from seven to seven and one half
pounds, boys weighing several ounces
more than girls. The skin is now
pink and as a rule is thickly coated
with a cheesy vernix. The fine downy
hair which previously covered its
body has largely disappeared. The
fingernails are firm and protrude
beyond the ends of the fingers. See
Chapter 11, The Newborn, for a
complete discussion of this topic.

HEREDITY

Heredity may be defined as the
tendency of an organism to develop
in the likeness of its progenitors. It
is, in other words, the transmission
of physical and mental qualities from
parent to offspring.

At the moment of conception the
male germinal cell combines with
the female cell, bringing together the
elements of the new life from the
two parents. We have seen that
the spermatozoon must convey the
material basis of paternal inheritance.
Similarly as has been stated above,
the ovum is the bearer of the maternal qualities inherited by the child.

In the germ cell of each sex is
contained all that the new individual
will inherit. In these two microscopic,
one-celled, complex structures lies a
potential man or woman who will
develop into a complete, complicated organism with a physical and
mental make-up not only characteristic of the ones from whom the person
originated but also of his forebears

as well. It is small wonder then, that
heredity is so little understood. This
still remains largely nature's secret,
one which man has spent countless
years investigating, with only a final
unknowing admiration.

Every living cell contains within
its nucleus, bodies visible under a
powerful microscope after special
staining; these are called chromosomes. The number of chromosomes
remains constant and definite within
each species. Each and every cell
of the human body contains 48
chromosomes in pairs, except the
mature egg or sperm which contains
24 of them unpaired. In ordinary cell
division during the development of
body cells the chromosomes divide
so that each cell has its characteristic
chromosome number. During the
ripening of the germ cell a reduction
division takes place which differs
from the usual cell division in that
one chromosome of each pair goes
to one cell and its mate to the
other. When fertilization takes place
24 chromosomes are contributed by
the egg and 24 by the sperm, so that
the new individual begins with the
usual 48 chromosomes.

The chromosomes are the bearers
of hereditary qualities. Each is composed of a large number of minute
particles called genes. Since they exist
in pairs, a set of genes is supplied
by each parent. Doubling of the
genes seems to be the main biological
reason for having two parents and
is a form of insurance, for if a gene
from one parent is defective it may
be offset by a corresponding good

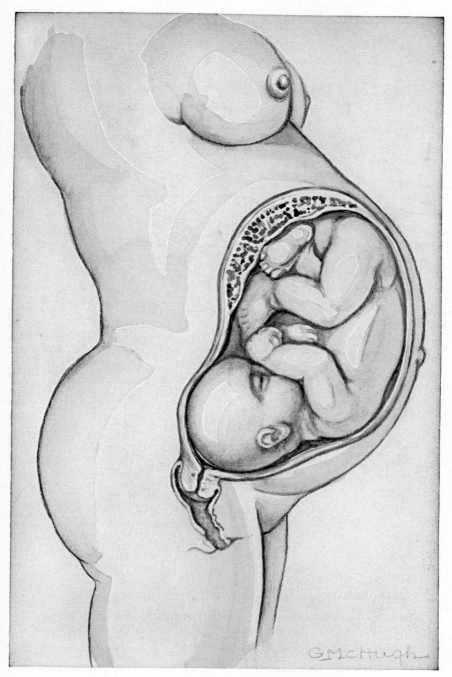

Fig. 13. Full-term fetus as it lies in the mother.

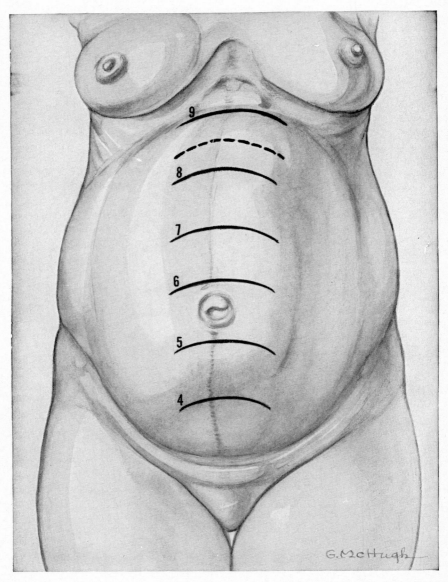

Fig. 14. The various levels of the uterus through the months of pregnancy. The broken line indicates the height of the uterus near term when lightening occurs.

gene from the other parent. The study of how the genes behave, how they interact and what characteristics they determine is a fascinating and complex subject known as the science of genetics.

Determination of Sex. One pair of chromosomes in the unripe germ cell is called the sex chromosomes. In the unripe male cell the pair is not identical, for one chromosome, designated X, is twice the size of its companion Y. In the female germ cell the sex chromosome pair always consists of XX. During ripening of the germ cell, as a result of the reduction division, half the spermatozoa will carry an X chromosome while the other half will carry the Y chromosome. In the female, however, all the mature eggs will carry one X chromosome. Fertilization of the ovum by a sperm cell carrying a Y chromosome will result in a boy (XY); fertilization by a spermatozoon with an X chromosome will result in a girl (XX). The sex of the child thus depends on whether a male-determining or female-determining spermatozoon fertilizes the egg. If this explanation is correct (and it is in accord with careful biological observations), it removes from the mother all responsibility for the sex of her child and places it with the father. Furthermore, since the facts indicate that male-producing and female-producing spermatozoa are present in equal numbers, it follows that there is practically an even chance that an embryo will develop into a boy or a girl. In any case the sex is decided at conception and can not be influenced after that time.

4

Mental Attitude and Beliefs

Popular opinion is the greatest lie in the world.
CARLYLE

Books written on the subject of the fallacies and superstitions of pregnancy make interesting reading. Nowhere in medicine is misinformation more prevalent and absurd, undoubtedly because the phenomena of conception, pregnancy, and childbirth are at once so ubiquitous, mysterious and miraculous.

Certainly science still has much to learn about conception and heredity, the factors affecting fetal development, the cause of the onset of labor, and other matters concerning reproduction. It is only in recent years that obstetrics has been elevated from the lowly status of a midwife's monopoly to the dignity of a scientist's art. It is little wonder then that the many beliefs which science has disproved have had wide acceptance for so many generations that, like any legend, they are difficult to supplant with truth. Not only do most of these beliefs serve no useful purpose, they often arouse undue worry and make miserable a pregnancy which would otherwise be pleasant.

Probably the oldest and most deep-rooted of the popular fallacies and superstitions is the idea that maternal impressions can alter the mind or body of the child in the uterus. The belief that a strange or ugly sight witnessed by a pregnant woman could affect the baby's mind or body dates from remotest antiquity. There is reference to it in the Bible, and the idea has been prevalent in the uncivilized and civilized worlds for centuries. Such famous authors as Goethe, Balzac and Shakespeare have used this idea as a basis of some of their plots, and great names of earlier medicine have credited it. But present scientific knowledge makes it certain that such a belief is ridiculous. We know now that there is no direct connection between either the blood or the nervous systems of the mother and baby.

Another common belief is that a seventh-month baby has a better chance to survive than an eight-month baby. How foolish this is! The best incubator in the world is the womb. And what do we do with the premature child? We place it in an incubator to give it its best chance to survive and develop.

Furthermore it is not true that stretching the arms high above the head, as in hanging curtains, is likely to produce a knot in the baby's umbilical cord. Knots do occur in the cord at times, due perhaps to its excessive length or to the turning of the child in the womb, but certainly not because of the activity of the mother.

The fact that a number of months pass before sex can be distinguished by direct examination of the fetus has led to the erroneous belief that it can be influenced during the early part of pregnancy or actually determined at will.

More than 500 theories have been offered to explain the relation and cause of the sex; nearly all of them have no reasonable foundation and are only of historical interest. The view that girls are derived from the right ovary, boys from the left, has long since been disproved, and deserves mention merely because many of the laity still believe it.

It was once believed that the sexes might be distinguished before birth by the number of heart beats occurring within a minute. In a general way, the action of this organ in females is somewhat more rapid than in males; and so it was thought that a rate of 144 or more indicated the female and a rate of 124 or less the male sex. But experience has taught that this rule leads to accurate prophecy in no more than half of the cases, or the same accuracy that random chance will give. No inquiry is more often submitted to the physician by prospective mothers than this, "Can you tell me if my baby will be a boy or a girl?" He cannot. The truthful physician will tell his patients that he guesses the sex of the babies incorrectly as often as he guesses it correctly. Normally, about 105 boys are born to every 100 girls and this ratio holds true regardless of seasonal variations and geographical divisions. Hence, if a physician guesses boys more often than girls, over a long period of time his correct guesses will be slightly greater than his incorrect ones.

The subject of superstitious fears forms a good introduction to a discussion of the mental attitudes of the expectant mother and father. For although it is true that a baby cannot be marked by maternal impressions, nevertheless serious emotional disturbance of the mother can react to the detriment of both mother and child. We know that undue mental strain can affect adversely the health of any person whether pregnant or not. That digestive, muscular, circulatory, and other physiologic disorders can arise from psychologic causes is now a well-recognized fact. It has become the basis of a separate study known as psychosomatics, which has been receiving increasing attention from the medical profession during the past decade.

From a physiologic viewpoint there are two main types of bodily functions—the voluntary and the involuntary. (These are purely arbitrary classifications, and may seem to the reader to be somewhat debatable in the light of the explanation which follows.) Movements of the extremities, eating, and even the act of breathing, although the latter is passive, are examples of voluntary activity. Variations in the blood pressure, movements of the intestines, and changes in the uterus are examples of involuntary activity.

We all know that various emotional stimuli can affect the latter type of function. Anger can cause an increase in blood pressure; fright, a rapid pulse; and extreme nervousness, a diarrhea. Naturally there are also other physiologic changes with each of these states. It is evident, therefore, that there is a definite and important interconnection among the the organs of the body, and an interaction that is intimate and complete. This union of bodily responses is affected by the dominance of the central nervous system, which controls in addition to all the nerves of the body, the glands of internal secretion, the action of the blood vessels, and the function of the vital organs—heart, liver, and kidneys.

The mind, though little understood, is known to be able to affect in any way any type of activity the body is capable of performing. Fear knows few bounds in its effect on the body. The voluntary muscles can become useless; legs that want to run, powerless; and the tongue can refuse to speak. Even more significant is the role fear can play in childbearing. The frightened, apprehensive laboring patient develops a state of tenseness that in some way raises the threshold of resistance of the passages in the birth canal,

thereby necessitating more frequent and powerful uterine contractions to effect delivery, with a correspondingly greater degree of discomfort and pain. It has been shown repeatedly that the well-informed patient adopts the attitude that labor is not a horrifying experience, but is nature's way of terminating the pregnancy. In the absence of fear this work can proceed more naturally and efficiently and with far less discomfort.

There is no better tonic than cheerfulness; it is beneficial to health. At any time there is nothing so harmful as worry, and particularly so during these months. Of course worry will not cause a baby to develop a neurotic temperament, as some believe, but it may affect the child and the mother physically by disturbing some of the functions of her body, possibly interfering with sleep or appetite or digestion.

The prospective mother should take cheerfulness as her motto. Cheerfulness will work wonders for her, her baby, and her home. She should keep in mind the overflowing happiness that a delightful, lively, rosy-cheeked baby will bring in a few months' time. The benefits to be derived from a well-balanced diet, plenty of fresh air, sunshine, rest, exercise, and pleasant diversions are most important to the pregnant woman. She should be sure to be outside for at least two hours a day. To sleep in the open air is good. And always the companionship of good friends is of inestimable value.

The mind should be kept busy—by reading light literature, perhaps, but this must not develop into a whole-day occupation, for exercise is also needed. Technical medical discussions should be avoided and such reading is easily subject to misinterpretation by the lay reader, and may cause undue worry over symptoms of minor importance. Her doctor is her best guide by far and she should feel free to call him.

Another recreation which might be mentioned here is card-playing. There is, of course, no harm in it. Indeed it is a wholesome way of relaxing if not abused, but it is fatiguing if indulged in too frequently or for too lengthy sessions.

Light housework is to be encouraged. If the patient has a sedentary position, as secretary or bookkeeper for example, she can work as long as the employer will allow, up to the day of labor, barring complications. Indeed such preoccupation makes a pregnancy more pleasant.

The Father-To-Be

The father-to-be should share actively with the doctor in the care of his wife while she is pregnant. His part is a larger duty than that of just paying expenses. He should know how important it is that his wife have proper medical care during her pregnancy. He should learn of just what such care consists. In some communities, classes for fathers, as well as for mothers, are held. The father-to-be should:

1. Put his wife under the care of a competent doctor early in her pregnancy and assure himself that the necessary examinations and and tests are made. In order to do this he must find out what these examinations and tests are. (See Chapter 1, Introduction.) He should encourage his wife to make maximum use of the care she is given, and should cooperate with her doctor by seeing that she follows all instructions for the health and protection of herself and the baby.

2. Arrange with his wife for her confinement and aftercare and help her in getting together everything she will need for herself and the baby. He should realize that many of the preparations for the baby's birth must be started as soon as the diagnosis of pregnancy is made.

3. See that his wife has proper rest and recreation. She should go to bed early and get up late, if possible.

4. Be a cheerful and patient comrade to his wife. He should talk over the coming of the baby with her and take an interest in her plans. He should relieve her as much as possible of worries and make her as happy as he can. She may not be her usual self at times, but he must overlook this.

In addition to the ordinary periodical reactions, pregnancy often produces depression, irritability, hypersensitivity, physical and mental indifference, and possibly impaired judgment. None of these conditions should surprise the husband; they are phenomena which, for the time being, his wife is quite unable to control. To bring an ovum of microscopic size to the highly developed infant it becomes, exacts a toll of all the mother's powers, mental as well as physical. She is in need then of particularly sympathetic treatment from her husband. His attitude should be patient, kind, and forbearing. He should take special care to avoid any remark or gesture which may increase his wife's irritability or bring about a collapse in her weakened condition. Although outwardly she may not appear to appreciate his efforts, she secretly notices everything her husband does, and values his kindness and understanding. In this way the bond between the husband and wife is made stronger.

"I give my husband three-quarters of the credit for my having such a lovely nine months," said one patient. "He has been wonderful to me." Would it not be gratifying if every wife could say the same thing of her husband?

5

Exercise, Travel, Hygiene and Clothing

Let her exercise be gentle walking, and the Heels of her Shoes low. In short, she must govern herself in these Exercises, rather to err in too much Rest, than in too much Exercise. It is impossible for me in this Point to be of the Opinion of all other Authors, tho' the whole World follows them in this evil and dangerous Counsel, who would have a pregnant woman exercise herself more than ordinary.

FRANCIS MAURICEAU, 1668

EXERCISE AND EMPLOYMENT

The benefits to be derived from exercise are improvement in the circulation of the blood, better appetite and digestion of food, better elimination of waste products of the body and more restful sleep. Women who have many household duties to perform need less exercise of other types than those without these chores. The amount of exercise that can be taken will be decided a great deal by how much the patient has been accustomed to before pregnancy. The important thing is to avoid exhaustion. Any violent form of exercise is absolutely prohibited. Housework is desirable for it keeps the mind occupied. There should be no lifting of children or heavy furniture. Reaching, as in hanging curtains, is objectionable only because of the additional strain imposed on the already stretched and tense abdominal mus-

cles. The idea that fresh paint is harmful to the pregnant woman is based on the fact that turpentine is toxic to tissues. To sleep or work in a recently painted room where no fresh air can enter may prove to be injurious, but there is no objection to the patient's painting or being around paint, provided that she does not inhale the fumes of turpentine in any degree of concentration. The prospective mother should learn to rest frequently, especially if she does housework. Fatigue here, as always, is to be avoided. An afternoon nap of an hour or so is beneficial and relaxing. There should be a minimum of 8 hours sleep in the 24; more, if required. A patient may sleep on her abdomen at any time throughout pregnancy—it will do the baby no harm.

Probably the most desirable form of exercise is walking; "Two miles

37

of air on foot" is a good daily rule. The walk should be taken during the hours of sunlight, for the sun's rays are beneficial. In the summer one must be cautious about over-exposure to the hot sun. About two or three miles is a fair average daily walk, this may be shortened some-what near the end of the pregnancy.

In the early months such exercise as swimming (not diving) in an easy manner, or golf, is permitted, whereas more active or violent forms of sport, such as tennis and horseback riding, are forbidden. No exercise, other than walking and light housework, may be done past the seventh month. Especial care must be taken at the time when the menstrual period nor-mally would occur.

A word should be mentioned here about injuries from such traumatic experiences as slipping on the ice or being involved in an automobile accident. Also, late in pregnancy, women tend to fall or trip because of the extra weight that throws them off balance—they become a bit clumsy. Only rarely will anything but a serious episode affect the baby, for nature has provided a scientific cushion. The baby bounces away from any impact, being suspended in amniotic fluid, which is almost in-compressible. If, following an acci-dent, the baby's movements are felt and there is no bleeding it is quite safe to assume that no harm has been done.

Shopping is a popular pastime for most women. During pregnancy, however, it has disadvantages. Noth-ing is so tiring as going about in crowded stores, so common sense should be used in this respect. When in a crowd, there is the added dan-ger of contracting infection, such as a cold or influenza. This is particu-larly true during the last weeks of pregnancy, when it is important to avoid all risk of infection.

TRAVEL

Certainly those who have lost babies before birth on previous oc-casions should avoid traveling when-ever possible. It should be kept to a minimum in all cases. It is during the first three and one half months that most spontaneous abortions occur. Here, as throughout the entire gestation, the vibrations, exhaustion and inconvenience of travel do no good. The hazard of being without proper medical care and facilities, should an emergency arise, also must be considered.

Formerly, automobile trips were absolutely forbidden, but there is a tendency today to be less strict in this respect owing to the improve-ment in roads and cars. The danger lies in traveling too far or at an ex-cessive rate of speed, thus produc-ing exhaustive muscular contractions which may even result in abortion.

Driving is a matter of personal discretion. A nervous person should never drive, particularly if driving is an effort. Long trips by train are to be avoided as much as possible, and if necessary should be undertaken under ideal conditions. There should be no rushing about or carrying of grips. With boat trips there is the additional hazard of seasickness.

Air Travel. Apparently no harm results from traveling by air. The airlines permit pregnant women to ride, and medical reports are not against flying.

CARE OF THE TEETH

There is an old saying, "For every child a tooth." This was based largely upon the popular belief that the fetus takes calcium from the mother's teeth and bones. While this occurrence may take place where the mother's diet is deficient in calcium and phosphorus, there is no danger of this when a proper diet is available or mineral supplements taken. Current medical thought holds that susceptibility to caries probably does not increase as a result of childbearing. Oral infection is often overlooked and should be investigated. The care of the teeth is most important during pregnancy, and the technic of proper dental hygiene should be completely understood and faithfully practiced. The teeth should be brushed from the gum toward the biting surfaces with a hard, short brush that has not been wet save with the dentifrice. The gums should be massaged with the brush to stimulate circulation of the teatlike processes which jut down between the teeth. Scouring of the teeth from side to side is harmful. The teeth should be brushed at least twice daily. The mouth should be rinsed with an alkaline wash several times a day. The teeth should be examined by a dentist early in pregnancy, as well as toward the middle and the end of pregnancy, and his findings and recommendations should be considered carefully. Necessary dental work may be carried out in safety. If anesthesia is required, the use of a local anesthetic is preferable. Oral infection should be treated.

It is opportune to stress the instructions on diet (see Chapter 6) giving the sources of calcium and vitamin D, which are essential elements for the proper nutrition of the teeth. The state of the gums and teeth reflect very closely the general health and nutrition; a focal infection may be the cause of miscarriage, kidney infection, etc., and may predispose to the development of a toxemia.

CARE OF THE HAIR

Falling of the hair is common during pregnancy. This should not cause undue concern, as the hair will soon grow again. Good care of the scalp is advisable; a shampoo will often be refreshing and stimulating. During cold weather, the hair should be dried thoroughly before going outdoors, to avoid the development of colds. There is no objection to a permanent wave.

SPECIAL HYGIENIC MEASURES

Baths. During pregnancy the skin must be given particular care. The patient is aware, by the changes in the appearance of the skin and her tendency to perspire, that the pores of the skin are more active than usual. They are throwing off extra wastes and poison, thus helping to relieve the kidneys of some of their new burden. To function properly, the glands in the skin must be free from accumulated wastes which may obstruct the normal outflow of secretions. To keep the skin healthy, a daily luke-warm bath is necessary. Care should be taken that the bath water be neither too cold nor too hot, the desirable temperature range being between 80° and 90° Fahrenheit. This provides for the elimination of noxious matter and gives to the body the beneficial effect of a fresh relaxed feeling and is neither stimulating nor enervating.

The bath may also be considered as a palliative remedy for nervousness and sleeplessness. The best time for the bath is in the evening before retiring, though the time is not of vital importance. To avoid colds one should not go outdoors for at least one hour after the bath during the cooler months.

After the eighth month tub baths should be discontinued and replaced by sponge baths and showers. The reason for this is that during the last few weeks of pregnancy labor may start any time and the tub bath might be the cause of child-bed fever either through introducing infection to the mother or by washing off the protective secretions with which nature provides her during the last weeks of pregnancy.

Care of Breasts. The circulation of the blood in the breasts must be perfectly free from any constraint, and for that reason any garment which presses down on the breasts is harmful. The breasts should be supported upward, and this can be achieved easily with a suitable maternity brassière.

It often happens that mothers are unable to nurse their babies because they did not give sufficient preparatory care to the nipples for this function. During the last four or five months of pregnancy they must be the object of special attention. The nipples should protrude so that the baby's mouth may have a strong enough grip to obtain the breast milk without effort. This is impossible if they are retracted. To shape the nipples they should be subjected to a daily massage and outward traction with the fingers. The skin of the breasts should be washed with soap and water daily, just as the rest of the body. Special precautions should be taken to remove the scales that frequently cover the nipples. These scales are due to drying of the discharge which normally exudes from the nipples during pregnancy. The nipples may be anointed daily with cocoa butter, cold cream or lanolin. Astringents, such as alcohol, should not be used because they harden the nipples, thereby favoring the formation of cracks which become avenues of infection.

Douches. Accompanying pregnancy, there is usually a whitish vaginal discharge, a leukorrhea. If it is excessive or in any way unusual, the doctor should be consulted. He may correct the underlying cause by a very simple measure. Washing high in the vagina with a bland soap, using the fingers, will usually suffice to provide good hygiene and protect against a persistent leukorrhea. Douches for this or any other condition should not be taken unless so advised by the physician, in which case the patient should make sure she obtains detailed instructions and understands the manner in which the douche should be taken. Close attention, however, should be given to local cleanliness, as the secretions may cause irritation.

For local hygiene, a mild soap or a mild antiseptic solution may be used as recommended by the doctor, or a solution of baking soda or boric acid (1 dessertspoonful to a quart of warm water). It is necessary to dry the parts thoroughly.

If the discharge is yellow or greenish in color, it is abnormal and very special care is necessary as such a discharge may be due to infection and be dangerous to the patient and to others in the home. Attention must be given to cloths used for local care as these may be infected. The hands ought to be washed thoroughly after local care.

Intercourse During Pregnancy. In healthy women sexual intercourse does no harm as long as the abdominal enlargement is not great. It is absolutely forbidden during the last six weeks of pregnancy since it may cause infection or stimulate premature labor. The patient should understand the danger. If she has shown a tendency to abort or to have premature labor, her physician will probably forbid intercourse at a much earlier time. It is unwise to have intercourse during the time her menstrual period would have occurred had she not become pregnant. That nature wishes to discourage intercourse during pregnancy may be inferred from the fact that many women lose their desire after the fourth or fifth month.

Care of the Bowels. A daily bowel movement is desirable although not absolutely necessary. A large amount of water taken throughout the day and the establishment of a regular hour aid in overcoming constipation. Dietary management for this condition is also important, with fresh fruits, stewed prunes, vegetables and cereals being used as natural aids to elimination.

In order to prevent constipation as much as possible and also to overcome it when it is present, the following rules should be observed:

1. An abundance of water should be taken throughout the day—at least eight glasses. This is particularly important during hot weather.

2. Every day an attempt should be made to have a bowel movement at exactly the same hour.

3. The diet should contain a large amount of fresh fruits and vegetables. Stewed fruits, especially prunes or figs, often prove valuable.

4. In some cases it may be necessary to inject from four to six ounces of warm olive oil into the rectum before retiring.

5. A glycerine suppository may be enough to stimulate the colon.

6. If the above measures fail, drugs may be resorted to and the

following are suggested. First, mineral oil should be tried, using a tablespoonful in the morning and again at night. If this is not effective, one may use milk of magnesia, the same dosage. If this proves unsatisfactory the doctor should be consulted. An enema should not be taken without consulting him first.

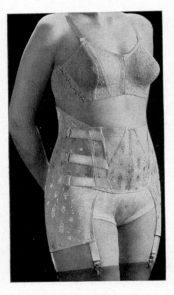

FIG. 15. Maternity corset and brassière (Spencer, Inc., New Haven 7, Conn.).

CLOTHING

Maternity Corset. It must be definitely understood that an ordinary corset should not be worn after the third month, as it may be harmful. However, contrary to what some believe, there is no harm in wearing the right type of corset for the purpose of support. It is more important for a woman who has already had one or more children to use a maternity corset than for a woman who is going to have her first baby. The reason for this is that most women who have given birth have some weakness of the abdominal wall and this requires support. Women who have a very flabby abdominal wall must wear a proper maternity corset constantly or they will have a good deal of discomfort, especially backache. Pressure from the baby, usually its hard head, upon the nerves of the pelvis can cause not only backaches and pelvic discomfort but also shooting pains down the thighs and legs. The complaints usually disappear when a supporting girdle is worn. This garment should be adjusted by an experienced person. Most of the up-to-date stores, understanding this fact, have specially qualified persons to fit the proper kind of corset and to make adjustments as required. There is no objection to the use of a two-way stretch; many patients feel more comfortable wearing one, getting only enough support to prevent fatigue or other symptoms.

Brassière. A well-fitting brassière should be worn. It should be designed so as to lift the breasts without compressing them, thus allowing good circulation. This circulation is important in the latter months to provide for the developing glands which are to be the newborn's source of nourishment.

Stockings. Wool, or silk and wool hose should be chosen for the cold weather. If light-weight stockings are preferred underhose or over-stockings should be worn for protection.

Garters. Round garters should never be worn because they will cause irreparable damage to the veins of the legs, not to mention the discomfort in the feet due to swelling caused by sluggish circulation. The thus creating a very tiring and even painful posture. Furthermore, as the abdomen continues to grow, there is a tendency to pull the body forward. To overcome this, the woman reflexly throws back her shoulders. If the woman wears high heels the body is pushed still further forward

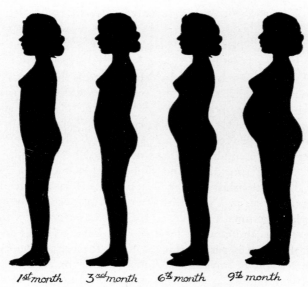

1st month   3rd month   6th month   9th month

FIG. 16. Diagrams showing posture changes as pregnancy advances (Zabriskie, Mother and Baby Care in Pictures).

suspender type of garter is the only suitable kind to wear. Almost all department stores and women's specialty stores carry them.

Shoes. An oxford shoe, with a low or medium heel, is the wisest choice. The harmful effects of high heels are not sufficiently recognized. The higher the heel, the more pronounced is the curvature of the back, and to save herself from falling she must throw her head and shoulders much farther backward. This causes a good deal of backache, discomfort in the lower part of the abdomen, and fatigue. Cramps in the legs can be due to improper shoes. During the latter months of pregnancy the feet spread and enlarge somewhat; slightly larger shoes must be worn.

6

Weight Gain and the Diet

Now good digestion waits on appetite and health on both.

SHAKESPEARE

The child in the womb depends upon the mother for his supply of food. Nourishment is not given directly from mother to child, because there is no open connection between them, but to emphasize the need for adequate nutrition, the maternal-fetal relationship is reviewed. The fetus lies in a sac filled with fluid which permits it to move about freely. An organ known as the placenta, or afterbirth is part of this sac. It is made up of myriads of small projections known as villi, in each of which is a small blood vessel. The villi dip into a collection of the mother's blood, and it is the coverings of these villi which extract from the mother's blood the food which the child requires. The nourishment which the villi take up is transported from the small blood vessels in the villi to large blood vessels which pass through a tube connecting the placenta to the child. This tube is known as the umbilical cord. It contains usually one vein and two arteries. The vein carries fresh blood containing nourishment to the child whereas the arteries carry blood containing waste products from the baby to the placenta; at birth this relationship between vein and artery is reversed. The impure blood is transmitted from the placenta to the mother's blood and the mother purifies it in the same way she cleanses her own blood, namely by eliminating the waste products through her bowels, kidneys, lungs and skin.

Since the connection between the mother and the child is so intimate, it is obvious that the child's development depends to a large extent upon the mother's diet and health. The child's growth is not entirely dependent upon the mother's food intake because if the diet is lacking in certain substances which the child requires, the substances in many instances will be extracted from the mother's tissues, usually to her detriment. A common example of this is the loosening and decay of the teeth during pregnancy when the mother does not obtain enough calcium and phosphorus in her diet to supply the baby's growth needs.

WEIGHT GAIN

During the first two and one half to three months, there should be little or no gain over the usual weight, perhaps a little loss at the very beginning. A patient may increase her weight thereafter a little less than two pounds a month during the second three months, which means a little less than one half pound a week, and during the last three-month period, three fourths of a pound a week. The ideal total weight gain is 18 pounds. The total weight that may be gained is still a matter of discussion. Most authorities agree that a 20 to 25 pound increase above the normal weight is the maximum amount that is desirable. This statement should be clarified. If the patient has an ideal weight before she becomes pregnant, then the number of pounds mentioned is permitted. On the other hand, if she is obese, a reducing diet is in order, and the net weight gain may be very little or none at all or the final weight may even be below that at the beginning of pregnancy. A thin, poorly nourished individual may be allowed a weight gain slightly in excess of 25 pounds. Each case is treated according to the conditions. Yet more important than the total amount gained is the rate which it is acquired. Sudden gains are likely to portend a metabolic disturbance and suggest an unfavorable condition, as such is often due to fluid in the tissues, which may not show quickly in a stout woman. Toward the end of pregnancy—the last seven to ten days —there is a tendency to lose a little weight.

The following summary can be made as regards weight gain:

The baby	7 lbs.
The afterbirth	1½ lbs.
Amniotic fluid	1½ lbs.
Increase in weight of uterus ..	2 lbs.
Increase in weight of circulating blood	1 lbs.
Increase in weight of breasts..	1½ lbs.

This totals 14½ pounds. The rest of the weight gain in an average normal pregnancy is due to a deposition of fat generally throughout the body, plus the retention of fluid in the tissues themselves. It can be readily seen, then, that the obese patient can actually lose weight with the proper dietary guidance, and a redistribution of her weight will result in the formation of the baby, the placenta, etc.

Generally speaking, those women who gain over 30 pounds place themselves in a group where the occurrence of toxemia is much greater. The significance of this can be appreciated by reading about toxemias in Chapter 8, Serious Complications. Also, women who gain excessively during pregnancy often have prolonged labors, due to the deposition of fat which diminishes the capacity of the birth canal.

WEIGHT OF BABY

Babies of excessive weight are not the result of heavy eating. There is no evidence to show that the amount of food taken by the mother greatly influences the size of the child. In former times diets were advanced to limit the child's weight. On the contrary, there is much to indicate that the size of the child is controlled in large part by heredity or by the duration of pregnancy, provided always that the patient has sufficient food to keep her in good condition. Observations made in Germany during the war, as well as much animal laboratory investigation, have shown that the weight of the offspring cannot be much influenced by the amount or character of the diet, except by a diet lacking certain vitamins. A sedentary life probably increases the weight of the child much more than does the type of food, provided always that the diet is balanced.

THE DIET

There is no more important time than during pregnancy for the diet to be sensible and well chosen. Granting that the fetus is, in effect, a parasite that takes from the mother's blood only that which it needs for its development, it follows that the pregnant woman who has sufficient and proper foodstuffs in her blood stream to supply the needs of the rapidly developing fetus will endure the strain of pregnancy with the minimum amount of damage to her body tissues. The mother should not assume that just because she appears to be strong she eats sensibly. She should remember that the majority of women with their first child are quite young, and that youth is so strong that nature appears kind.

A pregnant woman needs a diet sufficiently varied to supply the necessary amounts of proteins, fats, carbohydrates, vitamins and minerals, such as iron, calcium and phosphorus. It should be adequate to build up her tissues to full strength and meet her energy requirements without producing a marked storage of body fat. The nutritional value of the foods eaten is just as important as the number of calories ingested. This idea can not be emphasized too strongly. The minimum protein requirements must be maintained. A total of 1800 calories in a properly varied diet can contain all the essentials for a normal pregnant woman.

The diet should contain proper amounts of:

1. Proteins, to build and repair the mother's and baby's body tissues. They are found largely in such foods as milk and cheese, lean meat, fish, eggs, whole-grain breads and cereals, and some vegetables such as beans and peas.

2. Carbohydrates (starches and sugar), which furnish fuel for heat and energy and are found in large amounts in such foods as cereals, breads, honey, potatoes, sugar and rice.

3. Fats, which furnish fuel. Certain fats also contain vitamins. They are found in cream, butter, oils, fat meats and cheese.

4. Minerals, which form the chief building material for bones and teeth. These are found largely in milk, certain vegetables, and fruits. Vegetables should be cooked in as

little water as possible. The water in which they are to be cooked should be boiling when it is poured over them. After the vegetables are cooked, the water should be kept for soups and gravies in order to save all the minerals and vitamins in them that the mother needs. Iodized salt is better than the plain, for it satisfies the iodine requirements.

5. Vitamins, which are the sparks that keep the body processes active and regulate growth, are found in large amounts in milk and its products, egg yolk, meats, whole-grain cereals, vegetables, fruits and cod-liver oil.

Minerals are the chief building material for bones and teeth. Foods with high mineral content are desirable and probably are the best means of administering inorganic salts. These are found largely in milk, certain vegetables, and fruits. The best food containing calcium is milk or skimmed-milk products. Calcium is obtainable from beans, peas, and cauliflower in small amounts, but not sufficient to substitute for milk. Iron is obtainable from beef, liver, oysters and spinach, and less readily from eggs, potatoes, codfish, herring, tomatoes, peas, lettuce, dates, prunes, and strawberries. Iodine is usually necessary for a successful pregnancy but can be taken safely as a routine only by eating sea foods or using iodized salt.

With such a wide distribution of foodstuffs in various articles of diet, meals may be selected that are appetizing as well as wholesome. The expectant mother should not think that she has to eat more than usual because she is feeding the baby, but she should be sure to eat enough of the right kinds of foods. It is obvious that, in early pregnancy, the food requirements should not be greater than normal, but there is a misconception that after the first four months the baby as well as the mother has to be fed, that the enormous appetite that often develops must be satisfied for this reason. Overeating is bad for both mother and child. It makes more work for the kidneys, skin and bowels. The mother-to-be should chew her food well and eat slowly in order to enjoy her food and get the most possible good from what she eats.

Vitamins are of such importance that a brief discussion of them follows.

Vitamin A is essential to growth and reproduction. Sources of it are cream, butter, egg yolk, green and yellow vegetables and glandular organs such as liver. Most of the vitamin A preparations on sale are oils extracted from fish livers, especially cod and halibut.

Vitamin B is the antineuritic substance. The disease, beriberi, is due to a deficiency of it. This vitamin is growth promoting and also serves to stimulate the appetite as well as lactation. There are many fractions of vitamin B and one, B_6, is especially useful in certain cases in combating the nausea and vomiting of pregnancy. Vitamin B is widely distributed in the diet, especially in milk, whole grain cereals and fresh vegetables. No one with a varied diet need worry about not getting this in sufficient amounts.

Vitamin C. Insufficient consumption of this vitamin leads to a disease known as scurvy. The best sources are the fresh citrus fruits and fresh vegetables (the canned being 90 per cent as rich in this vitamin as the freshly squeezed juices and fresh vegetables). Cooking largely destroys the vitamin C content of these foods.

Vitamin D is popularly known as the sunshine vitamin. It is required for the proper development of bones and teeth and the prevention of rickets because it is necessary for the proper utilization of the calcium in the body. The best sources are sunshine, ultraviolet ray lamps, codliver oil, irradiated foods (especially milk) and viosterol. During the winter months, some form of this vitamin will be added to the diet, for the proper utilization by the body of calcium and phosphorus are dependent upon it. During the summer months the patient absorbs enough vitamin D from the sun to make such an addition unwarranted.

Vitamin E is found widely distributed in foods. There is no special food that need be taken for it. Its lack in some cases accounts for sterility and where a patient has frequent abortions vitamin E in large doses is prescribed.

Vitamin G (B_2) improves the general nutrition and is favorable to lactation and to the growth and development of the newborn. A deficiency of this vitamin can result in a skin, nervous and digestive disease known as pellagra. The source of supply is widely distributed in foods and is found especially in yeast, milk and fresh vegetables.

Milk is an invaluable food for pregnant women. If the patient has an aversion to milk or is allergic to it, calcium will be prescribed, but milk contains this and so much else that is beneficial that it is a "must" in the diet. Four glasses a day should be the rule once the diagnosis of pregnancy is established.

There is no reason why a normal pregnant woman should not eat more meat than before pregnancy occurred, notwithstanding an old superstition to the contrary. We now know that most pregnant women would do well to increase the amount of meat in the diet because of the great need for this body-building substance and the often low reserve present. Modern investigation has shown that much more harm is done by using much salt for seasoning and by eating highly spiced foods and articles known to be indigestible than by eating apparently unreasonably large amounts of meat and other protein foods.

Bulk to combat constipation, except in spastic constipation, as well as to supply necessary food, is best obtained from vegetables and fruits. The pregnant woman, depending upon her size, should eat daily one and one half to two pounds of vegetables.

Cutting down on sugars, sweets, and fats during pregnancy is a sensible precaution so long as there is enough fat and carbohydrate in the diet to furnish necessary energy. Desserts should be of fruits and not pastry. The pregnant woman should eat a grapefruit, two oranges, or an apple or two a day. Apples and prunes are usually well tolerated and aid considerably in elimination. Stewed and baked fruits are often preferable.

Fluids. At least 6 glasses of water should be drunk daily and in warm weather, because of greater quantities of perspiration, a minimum of eight glasses a day. An adequate fluid intake is necessary and seems to flush out the kidneys and prevent certain disturbances of these organs that are not rare at this time.

Cigarettes, Alcohol, Coffee and Tea. These are permitted only with the greatest moderation. Coffee and tea are harmless when only three or four cups are taken daily. Smoking is not to be completely condemned during pregnancy; those who ordinarily smoke should make an effort to curtail their consumption of cigarettes or, if at all possible, discontinue the habit. A maximum of ten cigarettes a day is allowed.

At dinner parties or social gatherings an expectant mother should be careful about the matter of drinking. The effects of alcohol may be harmful to the baby's delicate tissues, and will severely tax the mother's organs of elimination. In addition, it may engender a sense of false security and cause the mother to become careless. An occasional cocktail will cause no ill effect.

Pica. In some cases, pregnant women have a strong desire for foods out of season, or odd things. Chief among these are pickles, highly seasoned foods, and chalk (calcium). This perversion of appetite is known as "pica." Unless these foods disagree with the mother or cause an undesirable weight gain, the appetite may be indulged.

Summary. The chief reasons for eating and drinking the right kinds and amounts of foods and liquids during pregnancy are:

1. To provide materials for building tissue in the baby's body and replacing worn-out cells in the mother's body.

2. To supply enough of the necessary vitamins and minerals for both mother and baby.

3. To provide strength, heat, and energy for mother and baby.

4. To help keep the skin, kidneys, bowels and other organs of the body in order.

5. To prepare for nursing the baby.

In order to enable the patient to have a complete understanding of her diet, the caloric values of foods and suggested menus are presented below.

Food Values of Average Servings of Food *

Food	Approximate Measure	Calories	Protein (Gms.)	Calcium (Mgs.)	Iron (Mgs.)	Vitamin A (I. U.)	Thiamin (Mgs.)	Riboflavin (Mgs.)	Niacin (Mgs.)	Ascorbic Acid (Mgs.)
Milk										
Buttermilk	1 c.	84	8.4	284	.17	tr.	.096	.434	.24	2.4
Chocolate-flavored	1 c.	185	7.9	268	.17	221	.074	.394	.25	
Condensed	1 tb.	65	1.6	55	.04	86	.010	.078	.04	0.2
Dried, skim	5 tb.	198	19.6	715	.32	22	.193	1.080	.61	3.9
Dried, whole †	5 tb.	198	10.3	380	.23	560	.120	.584	.28	2.4
Evaporated	½ c.	178	8.9	311	.22	512	.064	.460	.26	1.3
Fluid, whole †	1 c.	168	8.5	288	.17	390	.098	.415	.24	2.4
Cheese										
American	1 oz.	106	6.5	236	.15	470	.011	.135	.05	—
Cottage	⅓ c.	97	18.4	79	.54	29	.019	.278	.09	—
Cream	⅓ pkg.	103	1.9	83	.05	619	.003	.039	.03	—
Fruits										
Apples, fresh	1 med.	81	0.4	8	0.38	114	.051	.025	.25	6.4
Apricots, canned	3 halves 2 tb. juice	122	0.8	14	0.41	1850	.027	.027	.41	5.5
Apricots, dried	10 halves	105	1.9	31	1.76	2675	.004	.058	1.19	4.3
Avocado	⅓ med.	201	1.3	8	0.46	220	.091	.114	.84	12.2
Bananas	1 med.	99	1.2	8	0.60	430	.090	.060	.60	10.0
Berries, fresh:										
Blueberries	½ c.	46	0.4	11	0.54	188	.020	.047	.20	10.7
Other berries	½ c.	46	0.8	25	0.63	224	.021	.049	.21	16.1
Strawberries	½ c.	42	0.8	29	0.82	61	.031	.071	.31	61.2

* Adapted from "Tables of Food Composition in Terms of Eleven Nutrients, Table 1," Bureau of Human Nutrition and Home Economics, U.S.D.A., in co-operation with National Research Council.
† Pasteurized

FOOD VALUES OF AVERAGE SERVINGS OF FOOD (Continued)

FOOD	APPROXIMATE MEASURE	CALORIES	PROTEIN (Gms.)	CALCIUM (Mgs.)	IRON (Mgs.)	VITAMIN A (I. U.)	THIAMIN (Mgs.)	RIBOFLAVIN (Mgs.)	NIACIN (Mgs.)	ASCORBIC ACID (Mgs.)
Cherries, red, canned in sirup	½ c.	86	0.6	11	0.30	430	.030	.020	.20	3.0
Grapefruit	½ sm.	126	1.4	49	0.86	tr.	.114	.057	.57	114.4
Grapes	1 large bunch	104	1.1	24	0.84	112	.070	.042	.56	56.0
Melons:										
Cantaloupe	½ med. slice	89	2.3	65	1.54	13167	.231	.154	3.1	127.1
Watermelon	6″ × 1½″	103	1.7	23	0.66	1953	.166	.166	0.7	19.9
Orange	1 med.	78	1.4	51	0.62	296	.125	.047	0.3	76.4
Orange juice *	½ c.	67	0.7	40	0.49	122	.085	.024	0.2	57.2
Peaches:										
Canned	2 halves or 3 tb. juice	160	0.9	11	0.85	959	.021	.043	1.5	8.5
Fresh	1 med.	51	0.5	8	0.60	880	.020	.050	0.9	8.0
Pears, canned	2 halves 2 tb. juice	75	0.2	8	0.20	tr.	.010	.020	0.1	2.0
Pineapple:										
Canned	1 slice	76	0.3	25	0.52	70	.061	.017	0.2	7.8
Fresh	1 slice; ¾″	50	0.3	14	0.26	113	.069	.017	0.2	20.9
Juice	½ c.	65	0.4	18	0.61	97	.061	.024	0.2	10.9
Plums, fresh	3 med.	76	0.9	23	0.68	473	.203	.041	0.8	6.8
Prunes, dried	4–5 med.									
Raisins	4 tb. juice	475	3.7	86	6.20	3005	.159	.254	2.7	4.8
Rhubarb, stewed	¼ c.	86	0.7	21	0.96	15	.044	.023	0.1	tr.
	½ c.	20	0.6	42	0.56	33	.011	—	0.1	9.9
Tomatoes:										
Canned	½ c.	25	1.2	13	0.72	1260	.060	.036	0.8	19.2
Fresh	1 med.	34	1.5	16	0.88	1606	.087	.058	0.9	33.6
Juice	½ c.	14	0.6	4	0.24	630	.030	.018	0.4	9.6

* Canned

Food Values of Average Servings of Food (Continued)

Food	Approximate Measure	Calories	Protein (Gms.)	Calcium (Mgs.)	Iron (Mgs.)	Vitamin A (I. U.)	Thiamin (Mgs.)	Riboflavin (Mgs.)	Niacin (Mgs.)	Ascorbic Acid (Mgs.)
Vegetables										
Asparagus:										
Canned	½ c.	18	1.4	17	0.85	510	.051	.087	.68	13
Fresh	6 stalks	13	1.1	11	0.45	500	.083	.088	.60	17
Beans:										
Green	½ c.	28	1.6	44	0.74	422	.054	.073	.40	13
Lima, dried	½ c.	147	8.9	29	3.23	—	.258	.103	.90	1
Lima, fresh	½ c.	106	6.1	51	1.86	146	.203	.113	.73	26
Cabbage, raw	½ c.	12	0.6	20	0.21	34	.030	.036	1.29	22
Carrots, raw	1; 4 in.	25	0.7	21	0.44	6600	.039	.036	.28	3
Chard, Swiss	½ c.	25	1.4	105 *	4.00	2800	.060	.130	.20	38
Corn, yellow	1 ear med.	38	4.7	12	0.64	243	.192	.189	1.79	15
Kale	½ c.	33	1.9	146	1.43	4901	.088	.23	.52	75
Lettuce	3 lg. leaves	10	0.7	35	0.63	923	.03	.04	.11	10
Okra	5–6 pods	21	0.9	43	0.37	392	.06	.05	.36	16
Peas, English	½ c.	61	4.0	13	1.14	408	.22	.11	1.26	16
Rutabaga	½ c.	50	1.3	67	0.49	403	.07	.07	.06	44
Spinach	½ c.	21	1.9	68	2.49	7819	.10	.20	.58	49
Squash, Hubbard	½ c.	44	1.5	19	0.60	4950	.05	.08	.60	8
Potatoes										
Irish	1 med.	102	2.4	13	0.84	24	.13	.05	1.44	20
Sweet	1 med.	203	2.9	49	1.13	12474	.16	.09	1.13	36
Beets	2 med.	46	1.6	27	1.0	20	.030	.050	.40	10
Broccoli	½ c.	21	1.9	74	0.7	20	.051	.119	.51	67
Cauliflower	½ c.	25	1.9	18	0.9	74	.082	.090	.49	57
Celery, raw	2 stalks	7	0.4	16	0.2	—	.009	.012	.09	2
Cucumber, pared	¼ med.	14	0.7	10	0.3	—	.040	.090	.20	8
Eggplant	½ c.	15	0.6	8	0.2	17	.039	.033	.44	3

* May not be available.

Food Values of Average Servings of Food (Continued)

Food	Approximate Measure	Calories	Protein (Gms.)	Calcium (Mgs.)	Iron (Mgs.)	Vitamin A (I. U.)	Thiamin (Mgs.)	Ribo-flavin (Mgs.)	Niacin (Mgs.)	Ascorbic Acid (Mgs.)
Onions, raw	1 med.	30	0.9	20	0.3	31	.019	.012	.62	6
Squash, summer	½ c.	19	0.6	15	0.4	260	.04	.05	1.10	17
Turnips	½ c.	31	0.9	35	0.4	tr.	.053	.053	.44	25
Eggs, Poultry, Fish, and Meat										
Eggs	1 med.	74	6.1	25	1.3	536	.056	.159	.05	—
Chicken, E. P.	¼ lb.	219	22.8	18	2.2	tr.	.124	.203	9.72	—
Turkey	¼ lb.	296	22.7	26	4.3	tr.	.136	.215	8.93	—
Fish:										
Cod	¼ lb.	79	20.6	20	1.0	—	.045	.056	2.60	2
Salmon, pink, canned	½ c.	87	10.7	35	0.7	42	.016	.094	3.38	—
Tuna, canned	½ c.	176	22.4	28	1.4	57	.032	.105	8.59	—
Beef:										
Chuck roast	¼ lb.	246	21.0	12	3.16	—	.136	.169	5.7	—
Rib roast	¼ lb.	313	19.7	11	2.94	—	.124	.158	5.3	—
Rump roast	¼ lb.	385	17.5	10	2.60	—	.113	.136	4.7	—
Hamburger	¼ lb.	357	18.7	11	2.81	—	.117	.170	5.0	—
Loin steak	¼ lb.	331	19.1	11	2.83	—	.113	.147	5.2	—
Round steak	¼ lb.	219	21.8	12	3.28	—	.136	.169	5.9	—
Lamb:										
Chops	¼ lb.	259	20.3	11	3.05	—	.237	.294	6.7	—
Leg, roast	¼ lb.	259	20.3	11	3.05	—	.237	.294	6.7	—
Pork:										
Bacon, broiled	2–3 slices	106	1.5	2	0.14	—	.071	.017	0.4	—
Chops, broiled	¼ lb.	329	17.5	11	2.83	—	1.175	.226	4.9	—
Ham, smoked	¼ lb.	434	19.1	11	2.83	—	.881	.215	4.3	—
Sausage	3, 3 in.	260	6.0	3	0.89	—	.123	.084	1.3	—

Food Values of Average Servings of Food (Continued)

Food	Approximate Measure	Calories	Protein (Gms.)	Calcium (Mgs.)	Iron (Mgs.)	Vitamin A (I.U.)	Thiamin (Mgs.)	Riboflavin (Mgs.)	Niacin (Mgs.)	Ascorbic Acid (Mgs.)
Veal:										
Cutlet	¼ lb.	180	22.0	12	3.28	—	.203	.316	7.2	—
Leg, roast	¼ lb.	210	21.6	12	3.28	—	.192	.305	7.1	—
Heart	¼ lb.	142	18.6	11	7.01	—	.610	.102	7.7	16
Liver, calf	¼ lb.	148	22.4	9	13.67	21696	.305	.316	18.2	35
Tongue	¼ lb.	228	18.5	40	7.79	—	.249	.305	5.7	—
Cereal Products										
Bread:										
Rye, light	¼ in. slice	68	1.8	0.1	0.22	—	.045	.011	.31	—
Wheat, enriched	¼ in. slice	60	1.9	13	0.41	—	.055	.035	.51	—
Whole-wheat	¼ in. slice	55	2.0	13	0.55	—	.059	.032	.74	—
Crackers:										
Graham	1 lg.	42	0.8	2	0.19	—	.030	.012	.15	—
White	1, 2"	25	0.6	1	0.09	—	.004	—	.04	—
Breakfast cereals:										
Corn flakes	½ c.	3.8	0.8	1	0.11	—	.017	.008	.17	—
Rice, cooked (½ c.):										
Brown	3 oz.*	267	5.6	29	4.13	—	.218	.038	3.45	—
Converted	3 oz.	261	5.7	8	0.53	—	.173	.030	2.85	—
White	3 oz.	261	5.7	8	0.53	—	.038	.023	1.05	—
Rice flakes	½ c.	22	0.4	0.5	0.05	—	.003	.002	.08	—
Rolled oats	½ c.	364	13.1	50	4.78	—	.506	.129	1.01	—
Shredded wheat	1 bisc.	100	2.8	10	1.03	—	.054	.038	1.13	—
Macaroni	¾ c.	587	21.2	36	1.96	—	.662	.130	3.42	—

* About ½ c.

Food Values of Average Servings of Food (Continued)

Food	Approximate Measure	Calories	Protein (Gms.)	Calcium (Mgs.)	Iron (Mgs.)	Vitamin A (I. U.)	Thiamin (Mgs.)	Riboflavin (Mgs.)	Niacin (Mgs.)	Ascorbic Acid (Mgs.)
Fats										
Butter	1 tb.	95	0.8	2	0.03	429	tr.	.001	0.01	—
Cream, 20%	1 tb.	31	0.4	15	0.01	125	.005	.021	0.02	.15
French dressing †	1 tb.	47	0.9	0.6	0.01	—	—	—	—	—
Lard	1 tb.	99	—	—	—	—	—	—	—	—
Margarine, fortified	1 tb.	95	0.1	0.3	0.26	469	—	—	—	—
Mayonnaise	1 tb.	101	0.2	2.7	0.14	29	.006	.006	—	—
Sweets										
Honey	1 tb.	99	0.9	2	0.28	—	tr.	.012	.06	1.22
Jams	1 tb.	91	0.2	4	0.11	3.5	.007	.007	.07	2.1
Jellies	1 tb.	91	0.1	4	0.11	3.5	.007	.007	.07	1.4
Molasses	1 tb.	55	—	63	1.54	—	.018	.037	.64	—
Sugar:										
Brown	1 tb.	34	—	7	0.23	—	—	—	—	—
Granulated	1 tb.	52	—	—	0.01	—	—	—	—	—
Various Desserts:										
Cake, plain	1/16 av. cake	98	1.9	19	0.60	—	.009	.030	.21	—
Cookies, Sugar	1, 2¼″ diam.	61	0.8	3	0.08	—	.006	.006	.07	—
Ice cream, Vanilla	½ qt.	279	5.3	176	0.13	718	.053	.253	.13	tr.
Pie:										
Apple	1/6 med.	266	2.9	11	0.19	—	.050	.040	.4	—

† With vinegar

DIETS

Normal Pregnancy Diet. This is a well-balanced 1800 calorie diet which will supply all the materials needed by the mother and baby during pregnancy—approximately 15 per cent protein, 25 per cent fat and 60 per cent carbohydrate. Each day include in the dietary:

1 quart of milk
1 egg
¼ lb. lean meat, poultry or fish (liver or kidney once a week)
2-4 servings of vegetables
3 portions of fruit—2 citrus fruits daily
1 serving potato
½ cup navy, kidney, lima or soybeans or peas or 1 ounce of cheese or 2 tbsp. cottage cheese or 1½ tbsp. peanut butter
3 slices 100% whole wheat bread or dark rye
3 tsp. butter or enriched margarine
3 tsp. sugar

Avoid fried foods, alcoholic and soft drinks, jello, ices, rich desserts— cake, cookies, pies, doughnuts, sweet rolls, candy, potato chips, popcorn, nuts, bacon and salad dressing.

Suggested Outline of Day's Diet

BREAKFAST

½ cup orange or grapefruit juice or 1 cup tomato juice
1 egg
1 slice whole wheat bread
1 tsp. butter
1 glass milk

LUNCH

½ cup navy, lima, kidney or soybeans or peas or cheese or cottage cheese
1 or 2 servings of vegetables
1 slice whole wheat bread
1 tsp. butter
1 serving of fruit
1 glass of milk

DINNER

¼ lb. lean meat, fish or fowl (broil, boil or roast)
1 serving of potato
1 or 2 servings of vegetables
1 slice whole wheat bread
1 tsp. butter
1 serving of fruit
1 glass of milk

1 glass of milk between meals or used in food preparation

SPECIAL DIETS

Low Caloric (Obesity) Diet (1200 calories)
The following foods should be avoided:

Fat meats—sausage, bacon, corned beef
Fried foods
Oils or salad dressings
Cream, gravies and sauces
Jams, jellies or honey
Alcoholic and soft drinks
Canned soups or rich stews
Jello, ice cream, ices, sherbets, puddings
Candy, popcorn, potato chips, nuts

Macaroni, rice, noodles
Cake, cookies, pie, doughnuts,
sweet rolls
Canned sweetened fruits

Suggested Outline of Day's Diet

BREAKFAST

1 average serving of any fresh fruit
Choice of:

1 thin slice whole grain bread
(may be toasted) or
1 small roll or
⅓ cup all bran

1 egg (boiled or poached)
Tea or coffee, as desired (no sugar
or cream)
1 level teaspoonful butter
1 glass skim milk

NOON AND EVENING MEAL, EACH

Clear stock soup
Choice of (in average serving of
2½ ounces):

Lean beef ⎫
Lean veal ⎪
Lean lamb ⎬ broiled, boiled or
White chicken ⎪ roasted
White fish ⎭

Two eggs
Cottage cheese
1 thin slice whole grain bread or
½ potato

Choice of:

2 servings of any of: asparagus,
brussels sprouts, cabbage, spinach, string beans, cauliflower,
sauerkraut
or
1 serving of any of: beets, carrots, turnips, squash, peas
Large serving of salad, composed

of any of the following: head
lettuce, tomatoes, string beans,
cabbage, beets, celery, carrots
Choice of fruit, as for breakfast
1 glass skim milk
1 level tsp. butter
In addition to the above: 1 glass
of skim milk between meals.
Saccharine may be used instead of
sugar; it has no caloric value.
A prescription for an adequate
vitamin product is given when the
patient is on a low caloric diet.

Anemia Diet. This is a well-balanced 1900 calorie diet for blood-
building. Each day include in the
dietary:

1 quart of milk
2 eggs or one egg and one egg
substitute
¼ lb. lean meat, poultry or fish
2 to 4 servings of vegetables
3 servings of fruit—2 citrus, 1
dried
3 slices of bread (100% whole
wheat)
1 serving potato
½ cup navy, lima, kidney, or soybeans or peas or 1 ounce of
cheese or 2 tbsp. cottage cheese
or 1½ tbsp. peanut butter
1 tbsp. molasses
1 ounce butter or enriched margarine

The addition of extra bread,
butter and peanut butter will increase the caloric content of the
above diet, if weight gain is desired.

Liver or kidney should be used
three or four times a week. Fruits
especially rich in iron are prunes,
apricots, raisins and peaches.

Preeclamptic Diet. This is an

1800 calorie diet for a limited period depending on the severity of the toxemia.

Each day include in the dietary:

3 glasses of milk
2 eggs or 1 egg and 1 egg substitute
½ cup cooked navy, lima, kidney or soybeans or split peas
¼ lb. lean meat or poultry
4 servings of vegetables (*no* canned vegetables)
3 servings of fruit—2 citrus fruit daily
1 potato
2 slices bread. (Home-made yeast bread made without salt preferred, or salt-free crackers)
½ cup cereal without added salt (oatmeal, rice or cream-of-wheat)
3 tsp. salt-free butter

Additions to the diet may be recommended by your doctor.

The following foods should be avoided:

Smoked or canned meat or fish
Corned beef, sausage, bacon
Clams, caviar, oysters, salt water fish
Cheese, except cream or cottage cheese
Salted butter or margarine, bacon drippings
Coconut, pickles, olives
Salted nuts, pretzels, potato chips, popcorn
Canned salted soups and vegetables
Oils or salad dressings
Fried foods, gravies, rich stews
Jello, ice cream, ices, sherbets, candy
Cake, pie, doughnuts, cookies, sweet rolls
Alcoholic and soft drinks
Salt, baking powder or baking soda should not be used in cooking; salt is not to be added at the table, not even in the smallest amount.

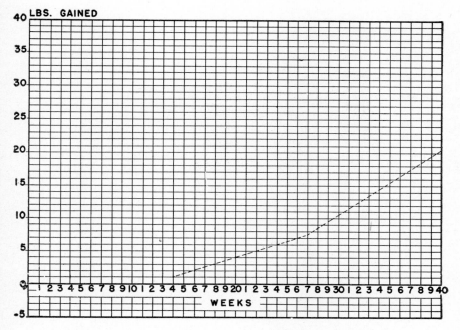

40 LBS. GAINED

35

30

25

20

15

10

5

0 1 2 3 4 5 6 7 8 9 10 1 2 3 4 5 6 7 8 9 20 1 2 3 4 5 6 7 8 9 30 1 2 3 4 5 6 7 8 9 40

WEEKS

-5

The above represents a chart showing the ideal weight gain. It will be noted that during the first three months of pregnancy there is no weight gain above the normal (0 on graph). Usually during the first six weeks of pregnancy there is a slight weight loss which is overcome during the latter part of the first trimester. During the middle three months, one-half pound a week is added and during the last trimester one pound a week gain is normal. Some patients will be able to keep the weight gain at this time as low as three-fourths of a pound a week in which case the total weight gain will be approximately 18 pounds.

It is suggested that this chart be used by the patient to tabulate week by week her own increase in weight, to compare her gain with the ideal.

It should be emphasized here that weight gain is an individual problem, and that the above curve is for the average patient—not for the obese or undernourished one.

7

Common Disorders

If all be well with belly, feet and sides,
A king's estate no greater good provides.
                                    HORACE

Nausea and Vomiting. Although a woman may be physically fit and may follow faultlessly a hygienic life, she may be affected early in her pregnancy by a wretched feeling of nausea and vomiting. Some experience these symptoms only in the morning while others are troubled throughout the day. This discomforting condition varies greatly in intensity with different persons. It may in some cases persist for as long as three months, but it is not without remedy and when recognized early can be controlled usually by proper diet and elimination. Small and frequent feedings at two- to four-hour intervals usually cure the mild cases, especially if fluid is not taken with meals. The more liquid the food, the more likely it is to be vomited. Water, especially, is not well tolerated. It is taken best at one hour after mealtime. The bowels may be regulated by the employment of mild laxatives. Antacids, such as sodium bicarbonate, magnesia, or citrocarbonate, frequently help. Either of two types of diet is suggested—one rich in carbohydrates, the other rich in

meat proteins. Both types achieve the result more by keeping food in the stomach than by virtue of the character of the food. However, the patient should not be kept too long on a diet which is inadequate in vitamins and proteins. Sedatives are somewhat useful.

Vomiting is less likely to occur if the mother:

1. Takes the right foods in small amounts
2. Has enough rest and exercise
3. Gets enough fresh air
4. Is not upset by grief, anger, worry or fright
5. Keeps the bowels and kidneys acting freely

When the nausea and vomiting are sufficiently annoying, a special regime as follows should be tried.

Before retiring two crackers are placed on a table beside the bed. Upon awakening the crackers are eaten without raising the head from the pillows. The patient should remain in this position for 20 minutes.

Breakfast. A light breakfast of, let us say, brown cereal and cream, toast and coffee. Butter should not be used on the toast; use marmalade, jelly or honey instead.

Midmorning. Crackers or toast with a glass of milk or cup of cocoa, tea or hot malted milk.

Luncheon. Vegetable soup with crackers, rice, green vegetable or fruit salad, bread or rolls.

Midafternoon. Crackers or toast with a glass of orange juice, grapefruit juice or lemonade.

Dinner. Lean meat, green vegetable, baked, boiled or mashed potatoes, rolls, tomato salad, dessert.

Before retiring, crackers or toast with a glass of milk or a cup of cocoa, tea or hot malted milk.

In case the vomiting persists and comes on frequently and does not respond to the above or to the various drugs that often prove beneficial, the patient will be sent to a hospital and treated according to one of the many recognized routines. Treatment by abortion is rarely necessary and is done only as a last resort.

Flatulence. Distention of the stomach and intestines with gas, a condition known to doctors as "flatulence," may accompany heartburn or appear independently. It is due usually to the action in the intestines of undesirable bacteria superimposed upon the circumstance that the pressure of the enlarged uterus and the very condition of pregnancy itself (the action of hormones) hinders the intestinal contents from moving along as rapidly as usual. Because of the latter fact, the primary consideration in the treatment of flatulence is regular evacuation of the bowels. At

the same time, care should be taken to avoid gas-producing foods such as beans, parsnips, corn, onions, cabbage, fried foods and sweet desserts. Some women find it helpful to have their vegetables puréed. For temporary relief, a level teaspoonful of baking soda (sodium bicarbonate) in one half glass of water is often helpful, as in heartburn.

Heartburn. Frequently during pregnancy there may be a burning or smarting in the pit of the stomach. This condition, heartburn, can often be corrected by drinking large amounts of water. Sodium bicarbonate (soda) in doses of one half to one teaspoonful in one half glass of water also generally gives relief. This medication may be repeated only 2 or 3 times daily and never should be used for more than two consecutive days, as excessive use will tend to alkalinize the blood. Milk of magnesia or cake magnesia may be substituted. Chewing gum sometimes helps. Other available antacids can be recommended upon the patient's request.

Leg Cramps. Cramps in the legs sometimes occur during the last months of pregnancy. They may come from muscle strain due to nature's effort to keep the body balanced as the center of the weight of the body shifts forward. Pressure on the nerves of the legs may cause cramps in the leg and foot muscles. Cramps may also be due to a vitamin or mineral deficiency, particularly a lack of vitamin B-complex, or to a lack of calcium. Cramps may come at any time while the expectant mother is asleep or awake. Relief may be obtained by:

1. Changing the position. This will generally relieve the mother-to-be quickly.

2. Bending the foot upward or pointing the toe downward.

3. Rubbing the cramped muscles (unless there are varicose veins over the cramped muscles) with olive oil or cold cream.

4. Wrapping the legs in hot or cold cloths, preferably part wool.

5. Lying down with the hips raised a little.

6. Taking vitamin B-complex.

7. Taking some form of calcium, as prescribed by the doctor.

Hemorrhoids or Piles. Many pregnant women are troubled by hemorrhoids. The usual symptoms are pain in and bleeding from the rectum while having a bowel movement. Hemorrhoids, sometimes referred to as piles, are a special form of varicose veins and they are always made worse by chronic constipation and straining at the stool. They are much more common in women who have had children than in those who are pregnant for the first time. It is important to eat the proper kinds of food and to go to the toilet at the same time every day. In addition, a tablespoonful of mineral oil should be taken by mouth, morning and evening. If the piles are swollen, ice compresses will help. If they do not readily return into the rectum they should be pushed back with a lubricated finger because of the danger of

obstruction and infection of these veins. If they cannot be pushed back or if they bleed frequently, the doctor should be notified. Suppositories and other medication will be prescribed as necessary.

Edema. This condition is a swelling of the body tissues. Usually it affects first the feet and ankles, especially during the last three months of pregnancy and in slight degree is very common and need cause no concern. It is more pronounced during the summer than the winter months.

The hands and face may become edematous—a usual sign of toxemia and one that must be reported to the doctor at once. A salt-free diet and other therapeutic measures will usually alleviate the condition.

Navel. It is not uncommon after the sixth month for the pregnant woman to notice that her navel instead of being indented has become flattened or even everted. This may give the impression that a hernia is forming. Actually it is merely a bulging due to the increased intra-abdominal pressure and will return to normal following labor.

Dyspnea. During pregnancy, especially the latter part of it, patients often complain of shortness of breath. This is known as dyspnea and can be due to any of several factors—changes in the circulatory system, variations in the contour and function of the heart, and an increase of abdominal pressure upward, preventing free movement of the diaphragm. There are certain circumstances where dyspnea is more acute, such as a large baby in a small mother or, more frequently, in the presence of an excess of amniotic fluid (known as polyhydramnios) as usually occurs in a multiple pregnancy. A multiple pregnancy necessarily imposes greater discomfort than a single pregnancy, the size of the abdomen being larger at term and also at an earlier date than in single pregnancy, causes proportionately greater pressure symptoms. Shortness of breath is often noted early in the pregnancy; heart disease or other constitutional variations as obesity must also be considered as a factor.

Pressure. Not only can the growth of the womb cause dyspnea from increased intra-abdominal tension but this very same development may mechanically affect certain pelvic and abdominal structures in a manner to upset the patient if she is not prepared for the occurrence. The intestines become crowded, enabling gas pockets to form, reflexly causing pain from the distended bowel. Change in position and the passage of flatus give relief. Rib pressure is very common late in pregnancy, the lower ribs taking the brunt of this new force; lightening consistently alleviates the discomfort. The liver, the spleen and the kidneys may be similarly affected, though to a lesser extent. After the seventh month, when the baby's head usually lies over the pelvic brim, the nerves which course over this area may be compressed, accounting for back-

aches or pains down one or both legs. None of these discomforts is serious; most of them develop gradually and are quite transient in nature. Mothers adjust quickly and soon learn to give such little heed.

Varicose Veins. During the course of pregnancy, the veins of the feet and legs should be observed, as these sometimes dilate, and if neglected they become varicosed or permanently injured. This condition can usually be traced to circumstances which have interfered with the free circulation of blood in the veins. Frequently the increased weight of the uterus in the lower abdomen is responsible; more frequently the wearing of such restrictive garments as round garters or a tight corset is the cause. Poor nutrition or insufficient rest in a recumbent position may be a contributing factor. Sometimes there is a hereditary tendency toward varicose veins, in which case the condition requires closer attention.

It is well worth a little care to prevent such a condition, for it can become very troublesome in later years. There are various sorts of bandages available to support the veins. They are not expensive and are very effective. Some bandages are made of silk crepe and some of cotton elastic mesh. Unresilient (nonelastic) bandages should not be used, for they will do more harm than good. Those containing rubber should also be avoided as they are hot and irritating to the skin. The bandage is applied from the instep to the knee, maintaining the same pressure on every turn. The patient will know whether it is properly applied from a feeling of comfort and from absence of swelling in the feet. It is neither beneficial nor practical to bandage above the knee. If the veins on the thigh are affected the only palliative remedy is to use an elastic stocking.

Nosebleeds. Frequently during pregnancy a nosebleed may develop. It is possible that pregnancy itself promotes nasal congestion and a tendency toward nose bleeding for it is a common occurrence without apparent cause. If the bleeding is scant and occurs only once or twice, it may be dismissed as unimportant. However, if it is profuse and persistent and tends to recur, it should be brought to the doctor's attention. The cause may be nothing more serious than the irritation due to conscious or unconscious attempts to clean the nose, but it will be the physician's duty to decide its significance.

Fainting. Many women faint in pregnancy or lose consciousness for a moment. They may become pale, but not necessarily so, and the pulse may or may not be affected. Such spells usually follow indigestion, but they may possibly be due to hormonal action or low blood pressure; in any case they are not uncommon in the first months of pregnancy. Smelling salts or aromatic spirits of ammonia are proper stimulants. Those who are subject to frequent attacks should carry some in a bottle to use when a

spell is approaching. Placing the patient in a position where her head is lower than the rest of her body usually results in a quick return to normal.

Some women notice that changes in position, especially sudden rising, tend to produce. dizziness and even fainting. If one recognizes this it is easy enough to avoid.

Drowsiness. The pregnant woman may feel drowsy during the first few weeks of her pregnancy. This is a common but annoying experience. It is probably nature's way of indicating the need. for an extreme amount of rest in order to adjust the mechanism of the body to the new condition. At least a couple of hours of sleep should be supplied during the day—one hour after the morning meal, and one hour after the noon meal.

Mental Unrest. Pregnancy may affect adversely the temperament of the expectant mother. She may experience a sense of depression, anxiety or irritability. In many of these cases this reaction is purely psychological, while in others a poor physical condition lies at the root of the trouble. The physician should be consulted and he will investigate the cause and treat it according to his findings. (Also, see Chapter 4, Mental Attitude and Beliefs.)

Salivation. Distress may result from an over-abundance of saliva, which may or may not be associated with nausea and vomiting. Where it is frothy and thick the condition is called "cotton spitting." For relief baking soda may be tried in small doses—one teaspoonful every three or four hours. If not effective after two days, any further treatment should be sought from the doctor.

Fetal Movements. At times over-activity of the baby may result in insomnia; and occasionally fetal movements may be actually painful. The prescription in such a case is a mild sedative which serves not only to relieve the mother but also to quiet the baby. The activity of the fetus is not only from movement of its extremities but also is due to rotations of the trunk and changes in its polarity (from head down in the pelvis to buttocks down and vice versa). It is not unusual for the mother to notice jerking movements by the fetus as though it were hiccoughing; strangely enough, that is exactly what it may be doing.

Lightening. At about six weeks before the end of pregnancy in most primiparas and in women with well-preserved abdominal muscles, the baby's head drops deep into the pelvis, permitting the uterus to displace itself downward, a process known as "dropping" or, technically, "lightening." It often causes a sensation of pressure on the rectum and is also associated with a desire to urinate frequently. Lightening gives the patient a sense of relief in some respects for there is freer breathing and less intestinal compression, and an increase in the capacity of the abdomen.

Allergy. Allergic diseases are occasionally aggravated by pregnancy, especially asthma. Patients who have hay fever and asthma should not receive immunizing injections because of the possibility of abortion.

Flushes and Sweats. Though it is unusual for a woman who is pregnant to complain of these symptoms they do occur frequently enough and without any untoward effects to be called normal. The flushes and sweats usually are of short duration and may come anytime during pregnancy. Sweats are a rather common complaint during the time of the early puerperium.

Numbness and Tingling. Some women experience numbness or tingling of the fingers and less often of the toes during pregnancy. Typically, this begins in the second trimester and is the result of a circulatory deficiency. As the baby grows there is an increasing demand for a larger blood supply by the uterus. As a consequence the circulation to the extremities may be relatively sluggish, and the above symptoms are noticed. This is certainly not a serious condition and can be overcome by frequent massage to the affected areas and also by applying heat in the form of hot water.

8

Emergencies and Serious Complications

*If the blind lead the blind, both shall fall into the
ditch.* MATTHEW

There is a tendency among women to regard some of the disturbances which come during the childbearing period as a necessary part of pregnancy. There is no truth in the old saying that, "A sick pregnancy is a safe one." There is no possible advantage in enduring any pain or distress that can be prevented by safe means; much harm may result from neglect. *Symptoms of trouble should not be disregarded!*

EMERGENCIES

If *any* of the following symptoms appear an immediate report should be made to the physician.

1. Bleeding (not to be confused with the "bloody show")—see Chapter 9
2. Labor contractions are well established. (See discussion under Labor, p. 79)
3. Bag of waters breaks
4. Chills and fever
5. Stubborn constipation
6. Shortness of breath or inability to sleep unless the head is elevated on a few pillows
7. Failure to feel the baby move after it has been definitely felt for a while
8. Manifestations of a toxemia

a. Sudden appearance of headaches, dizzy spells, persistent vomiting, spots before the eyes or epigastric pain
b. Sudden swelling of the feet, ankles, hands, eyelids or face
c. Rapid gain in weight
d. Diminished output of urine
e. Blurred or double vision, or spots before the eyes

These are nature's red lights, her danger signals. Mothers should know the signals and heed the warnings. In order that the patient may better appreciate the importance of these emergencies, a short discussion of them is worth while.

Bleeding during pregnancy is significant. During the early months of pregnancy it usually means a threatened abortion (a tendency toward miscarriage—see below). During the last three months bleeding is of great consequence and can *never* be safely neglected. When caught early, little harm should result, but if there is a delay, serious damage, both to the mother and the baby can ensue. Save everything passed—blood, blood clots, as well as soiled towels and sheets, so that an accurate estimate of the blood loss and the type of tissue can be made.

Do not let the lack of pain deceive you. Call at once!

Regular Pains. This topic is discussed fully in Chapter 9, The Labor, p. 76.

Breaking of Bag of Waters. This is treated under The Onset of Labor in Chapter 9, p. 79.

Chills and fever can be evidence of such general infection as influenza or pneumonia or many other specific diseases, but during pregnancy they may indicate pyelitis or cystitis. These inflammations of the urinary tract are quite common, and must, like any ailment, have early treatment. A high fever lasting a day or longer may produce premature labor. Report the presence of chills or fever or any evidence of infection.

Stubborn constipation is more common early in pregnancy than later. When present it should be reported so that a method of overcoming it safely can be prescribed. Cathartics and enemas endanger the pregnancy.

Dyspnea (Excessive Shortness of Breath). Pregnancy is not without its discomforts, and shortness of breath due to enlargement of the uterus has been mentioned already. If this is exceedingly troublesome or if sleep is impossible without pillows due to shortness of breath (often a sign of poor heart action), the doctor should be notified.

Absence of Fetal Movements. Once the baby is felt (quickening) the mother is constantly aware of its presence and normally notices periods of inactivity. An expectant mother should not begin to worry when she merely has failed to feel the baby's movements for a day, for this often is experienced when the baby is quite healthy. Nevertheless, should the baby not be felt for two or more days, the doctor should be so advised. He should be able to reassure the mother immediately, if the pregnancy has passed the sixth month.

The signs that the baby may have died are cessation of any movement, sometimes a feeling of weight in the lower part of the abdomen, often a cold, chilly feeling in this region, a rapid reduction in the size of the abdomen, perhaps a chocolate-colored discharge, softening of the breasts, a sensation of nausea or digestive disturbances, and a loss of body weight.

Toxemia. This is a condition occurring only in pregnancy, and rarely during any but the last three months. It is accompanied by an elevation of the blood pressure, swelling of the body (edema), the presence of albumin in the urine, and certain other symptoms based on the physical changes within the body. There is an excessive and often rapid gain in weight which accounts for the edema, noticed usually in the ankles and feet first, next in the hands and face, then the body. Headaches, dizziness, spots before the eyes and blurring of the vision are due to blood vessel changes, high blood pressure, and edema of the brain. Still later, the patient has sharp pains in the pit of her stomach. She vomits frequently and the urine output is diminished (less than three pints daily is serious). At this stage the most serious form of toxemia (eclampsia) is imminent. Good prenatal care and early attention to symptoms prevent eclampsia! Eclampsia is attended by convulsions and coma. The outlook for the mother and baby is grave. It is one of the three most common causes of maternal death; infection and hemorrhage are the others.

Thus, when any of the complaints mentioned under manifestations of a toxemia persist, inform the doctor at once. A special plan for such cases will be advised, according to the condition. Diet, sedation, medication and hospitalization, if necessary, will form part of the treatment.

Obstetrical Complications of Pregnancy

Abortion. In taking a history the doctor will inquire if the expectant mother has ever had an abortion. The lay person looks upon this word as implying a criminal procedure, whereas the medical profession uses it interchangeably with the word "miscarriage" with a preference for the former term. Medically speaking, it means interruption of pregnancy before the fetus is viable, i.e., before it is capable of extra-uterine existence—through the 28th week.

There are several types of abortion. Those due to natural causes are known as spontaneous abortions. Therapeutic abortions are those effected for the protection of the

mother's health, to prevent a disease, such as tuberculosis or heart trouble, from progressing and impairing permanently her physical well-being. When a physician feels that it is his duty to advise interruption of a pregnancy, first he must get the approval of at least one consultant and in some states two.

Complete, Incomplete, and Threatened Abortion. When an abortion occurs and all the products of gestation are expelled, we speak of it as a complete abortion. If a part of these products is retained, then there is the problem of an incomplete abortion which usually requires a minor operation (scraping of the uterus). Not rarely a patient pregnant only a few months begins to bleed and/or to have a menstrual type of cramps. This is an indication that she may abort and is called a threatened or impending abortion. Such is not to be confused with the slight staining that many women notice at the time of the first missed menstrual period. This is known as implantation bleeding and is due to the fertilized egg's burying or implanting itself in the lining of the uterus. As it does so, a small blood vessel is penetrated, and a few drops of blood escape and eventually appear externally.

Spontaneous and Habitual Abortion. A tremendous number of abortions occur for apparently no reason at all, and come under the heading of spontaneous abortion. The underlying cause is very often a defect in the egg, so that if it had not occured a deformed baby might have been born. Nature uses this way of sparing the family much grief, so one may find consolation in this knowledge should the accident ever occur. When the experience is undergone several times by the same individual, we classify her as a habitual aborter. It is indeed unfortunate that a specific cause, as a misplaced womb or cystic ovary, is not usually present, for in such cases the future is full of promise, as the condition can be corrected. At times we can overcome this tendency to abort by very simple measures, but this is just a small percentage of cases. Undoubtedly dietary and endocrine deficiencies—constitutional factors—play a role and success can only be obtained when this condition is fully studied, understood and treated accordingly.

Most spontaneous abortions occur during the second and third months; thereafter, the likelihood of the accident is much less. Commonly the first symptom is slight bleeding, followed by a menstrual type of cramps. There may ensue for several weeks a red-brown discharge and then a bright red flow, followed by the passage of clots and severe cramps, the latter being uterine contractions by which the products of conception are expelled. When everything within the uterus is passed the patient soon stops bleeding. But often a part of the placenta or embryo is retained and bleeding will not cease until the womb is scraped (the incomplete type of abortion). Once bleeding begins, the outlook for the pregnancy is not good. In any event, all clots

and tissues passed should be saved for the doctor to examine.

The treatment of threatened and habitual abortion is somewhat similar and should be understood by the patient so that in appreciating its importance she will co-operate completely and follow the doctors orders meticulously.

In the treatment of threatened or impending abortion, the most important factor by far is rest. This encompasses more than the word itself implies for it includes all forms of quiescence and repose for the body and mind in general and the womb in particular. Thus when symptoms appear, complete cessation of activity through bedrest and sedation is essential but this is not enough. There must be freedom from worry (emotional disturbances can effect the uterus, as is mentioned elsewhere) and lastly, drugs which prevent uterine activity are prescribed. More specifically, it is advisable for the patient to remain in bed until one week after the last day of bleeding or three days after all painful cramps have disappeared if there has been no bleeding. Reappearance of either symptom contraindicates resumption of activity. For the duration of her pregnancy the patient will have to restrict her activities, avoiding heavy housework, all forms of exercise but walking, marital relations and of course emotional strain. In addition to this she must remain in bed a few days before, during and after the time of her calculated menstrual periods, when a good percentage of abortions take place. Furthermore, she will continue taking certain prescribed medicines throughout most of the course of her pregnancy.

In cases of habitual abortion the treatment likewise is meticulous and specific. Such patients often present themselves to the doctor in their first few weeks of pregnancy being aware of their own deficiency or weakness, and prophylactic measures can be instituted early. The objective is to render the womb an incubator in which the fetus can develop and grow without trauma or outside stimulation and in a tranquil atmosphere. The nutrition must be adequate and above all well balanced. To attain this end the patient must spend much of her time in bed, especially near and at her anticipated menstrual periods. Exercise other than short walks is forbidden, intercourse is excluded, travel, and heavy or prolonged housework are to be avoided. Emotional disturbances are to be held injurious by the patient, her husband, relatives and friends, and everything must be done to maintain a cheerful and optimistic mental attitude. Lastly, adequate nutrition must be supplied and this means just that and no less. Thus the caloric intake must be well adjusted, the correct minerals (especially calcium, phosphorus, iron and iodine) should be sufficient, all the vitamins (particularly E and D should be given in large doses) and the hormones known to have a beneficial effect must be taken in adequate amounts. These include

thyroid at least and probably progesterone and estrogen as well; the latter two depending upon the blood levels and other factors to be determined by the physician.

By way of summary, it must be emphasized that the chances for a threatened or habitual abortion terminating successfully are limited and that the most important single factor in the treatment is adequate rest, without which all other forms of treatment are a waste of effort, time and expense.

Criminal Abortion. By far the largest group of abortions are those done outside the law for social, economic or other reasons and are known as illegal or criminal abortions. Hundreds of women die annually and thousands more are crippled by illegal attempts to interrupt an early pregnancy. There is no drug known to the medical profession which will produce successfully an abortion. Most drugs recommended by friends or druggists serve only to cause nausea, vomiting and severe diarrhea, and, at best, bleeding which requires a minor operation to control. Some drugs used for this purpose contain quinine or other substances that are toxic to tissue in unusually large amounts. Thus it follows that if huge doses of such drugs are taken and the uterus is *not* emptied, there is the danger that harm could come to the sensitive nervous system of the fetus, resulting in such a tragic condition as deafness or blindness. Those who perform abortions (other than the therapeutic abortions mentioned above) work outside the law and under the handicaps of poor assistants, poor anesthesia and poor equipment. It is little wonder then, that so many women

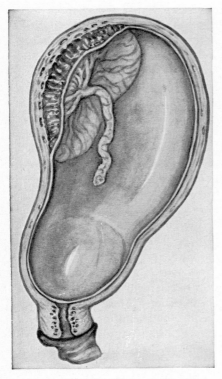

Fig. 17. The placenta lying in its normal position within the uterus.

die of infection and/or hemorrhage or suffer "female trouble" the rest of their lives because of criminal instrumentation.

Premature Birth. The termination of gestation after the baby is viable (28 weeks) but before term is known as premature birth. Such a baby is capable of living outside the mother's body but its chances of survival are not so good as if it had had the benefit of a longer stay in the womb. Thus prematurity itself, attended by low resistance to infection, changes in temperature, etc., accounts for the lower survival rate in this group of babies.

The causes of premature birth are varied and usually unknown, but contributing factors are accidents, overwork, and abnormal conditions in the mother, such as toxemia or syphilis. Prenatal care does much to prevent early labor. For further discussion, see Chapter 11, The Newborn.

Ectopic Pregnancy. A pregnancy that occurs outside the uterine cavity is known as an ectopic pregnancy. In this type of pregnancy the fetus usually lies in a fallopian tube, in which case it is known as a tubal pregnancy. Occasionally the embryo grows in an ovary, or in the abdominal cavity outside the uterus; these are called ovarian or abdominal pregnancies, respectively.

Ectopic pregnancies can be the source of serious complications and when diagnosed usually require immediate surgery because of the ever-present danger of rupture and hemorrhage; fortunately, they are rare in occurrence. When treated early, a favorable outcome for the mother can be expected.

Placenta Previa and Premature Placental Separation. Bleeding at any time during pregnancy is serious and should be given every consideration. During the last three months it has special significance. When not treated early or when improperly managed it may lead to fetal death and, not rarely enough, the loss of a mother.

The two commonest conditions attended by bleeding late in pregnancy are placenta previa and premature placental separation. The former is a condition where the afterbirth lies low instead of high in the womb. As the cervix opens up in labor, or due to the normal changes in the uterus that occur in the last trimester before labor, the placenta starts to separate from the uterus, leaving the vessels open to bleed. In premature separation, as its name implies, the placenta is in its normal location but because it is diseased, or for some unknown reason, it comes loose from its attachment before the baby is born and bleeding follows.

The treatment of these emergencies requires great judgment and skill. The patient must be transported to a hospital in an ambulance at once. She must be typed for a blood transfusion, the delivery room held in readiness for a major operation, and the patient examined vaginally. The exact handling of the case following this preparation and examination depends upon many technical points. It is enough for the patient to be familiar with the foregoing so that she will call her doctor at once and give him every opportunity to institute the best treatment to insure the safety of his patient. Early care means a happy outcome.

MEDICAL COMPLICATIONS OF PREGNANCY

Heart Disease. Since pregnancy usually takes place in young or rela-

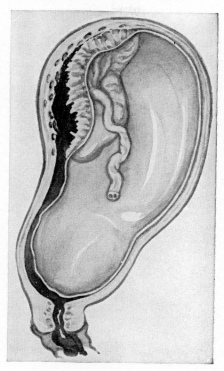

FIG. 18. Premature placental separation. Note the blood between the placenta and the uterine wall, separating the former from the latter thus interfering with the fetal circulation.

tively young women, and since heart disease is more a disease of middle and old age, it follows that the problem of heart disease in pregnancy is not a common one. Important here is the history of the patient; we must know what illnesses have affected her in the past and whether or not her heart was involved—and if it was, how extensively. The examination, of course, will be reveal-

unfavorable history does exist, the meticulous observation and care of the patient is constantly required. Fortunately, cardiac patients have

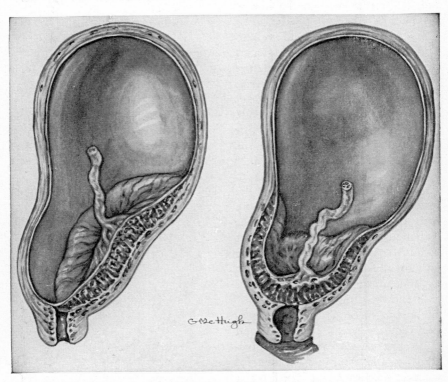

FIG. 19. Placenta previa. The placenta lies low in the uterus, in contrast to its normal location in the fundus, as shown in Figure 16. On the right the placenta lies directly over the cervical canal and blocks completely the passageway from the uterus to the lower birth canal, the so-called central type of placenta previa. On the left is seen a less serious form of this condition.

ing. In doubtful or serious cases, a specialist in the field will be called in consultation. The patient who has never had cardiac decompensation (heart failure) need not fear that it will happen during pregnancy or labor. On the other hand, where an

easy labors. The patient is spared as much pain and discomfort as possible and the baby is delivered using forceps to avoid the "bearing down" efforts of the second stage of labor. Rarely is a cesarean section done; when it is, sterilization at the same time is given consideration in certain patients.

Tuberculosis is a common affliction among women of the childbearing age. Its presence may contraindicate a pregnancy. Early in pregnancy a routine chest examination, including an x-ray or fluoroscopic study is made, thus permitting early diagnosis of the disease, even before symptoms appear. Such a complete study gives the doctor his greatest opportunity to aid the patient not only to improve her general health but to bear a child successfully and also to protect the health of the child.

Diabetes. This is no longer a serious complication of pregnancy, for when the condition is controlled by the use of insulin and diet, or diet alone, the outlook is excellent for the mother and brighter than ever for the baby. It is wise in most cases to have a specialist in consultation throughout the pregnancy and labor. Cesarean section is given serious consideration when this condition is present.

Anemia. During the course of pregnancy many mothers develop some degree of anemia. To prevent this condition it is necessary that the diet be rich in iron. The best sources from which to obtain this food element are liver, kidney and vegetables. If additional iron or blood forming stimulant is necessary, as is often the case, the doctor will prescribe appropriate medication. When taking an iron preparation one can expect the stool to have a dark tarry appearance.

Syphilis. Frequently the physician is greatly surprised when a positive Wassermann or Kahn reaction is reported from the blood serum of a woman who appears absolutely normal. There is a disagreement as to what should be done in such event unless the reaction is well pronounced. Usually a carefully performed positive test indicates syphilis. In case of doubt, it is safer to treat for the disease than to omit this wise precaution. Women who have had syphilis which has been treated until a negative Wassermann has been obtained should always be treated during pregnancy. Some women should be treated "on suspicion" when the history suggests syphilis. Such therapy does not cause abortion or premature labor, but tends to prevent these as well as to prevent or cure syphilis in the fetus. A Wassermann of the husband and any children in the family should be taken when the patient has a positive reaction. False positives occur occasionally, due either to a laboratory error or because pregnancy changes the blood in a way that it results in such a reaction. If the father of the baby has syphilis but the mother has not, the baby will be disease free.

Gonorrhea. This is the commonest of the venereal diseases and unfortunately is not rare even during pregnancy. At one time, before the disease was so quickly diagnosed and before every newborn's eyes were treated with silver nitrate, gonorrheal infection of the eyes was a common cause of blindness. The chief symptoms are a persistent greenish, purulent, irritating vaginal discharge often associated with urinary discomfort and fever. Checked early the unpleasant effects can be completely avoided and childbed fever or subsequent gynecologic difficulties prevented.

The diagnosis is now readily made on the basis of the physical findings and a laboratory analysis of the discharge. The treatment is begun as soon as a diagnosis is established, and consists of chemotherapy. This gives a most remarkable, rapid and dramatic cure.

Urinary Tract Infection. This is not a rare complication of pregnancy and occurs most often during the late middle and latter part of pregnancy. The bladder, kidneys, and tubes connecting these organs may be involved simultaneously, or individually. Cystitis, pyelitis and ureteritis are the scientific terms used to indicate inflammation of these organs, respectively. The exact cause is not always discoverable but it is felt that urinary stagnation, quite characteristic of pregnancy, is a factor, and that a previous infection or current focus of infection (teeth, tonsils, appendix, etc.) may be important causes. The symptoms are variable and include fever, back pain, chills, and pain with urination. Examination of a urine specimen shows the presence of pus. Treatment is quite satisfactory; chemotherapy and the removal of any focus of infection completely solve the problem.

Thyroid Disturbances. Sometimes during pregnancy the function of the thyroid gland is disturbed. This gland may be overactive or deficient. If it becomes hyperactive, the condition may show itself by extreme nervousness, some slight tremor of the fingers, a rapid pulse, weakness, loss of weight, with or without protrusion of the eyes and with or without enlargement of the gland. Goiter is particularly prevalent in certain sections of the country where there is an insufficient amount of iodine in the food. Iodized salt is a preventive, and it is also effective in treatment. An occasional meal of seafood is one way of obtaining iodine naturally, as is also the use of iodized salt.

If the thyroid gland is underactive, the patient, instead of showing marked nervousness, may become dull and disinterested, and may rapidly gain weight. Vomiting is occasionally traceable to this cause. The doctor can diagnose malfunction of the gland readily from his physical examination and from a basal metabolism test. An extract of this gland will immediately overcome any deficiency, not only improving the patient's health, but making sure that the baby will be free from a comparable condition.

German Measles. There is increasing evidence that a woman who acquires german measles when she is less than three or four months pregnant is likely to give birth to a baby that is defective in some way. The question of a therapeutic abortion under this circumstance must be given consideration.

9

The Labor

The greatest battle that ever was fought
Shall I tell you where and when?
On the maps of the world you will find it not:
It was fought by the Mothers of Men.
JOAQUIN MILLER

The sentiments so vividly and beautifully expressed in the poem above were poured from a sympathetic heart and could well refer to the pain suffered in days past by women in labor.

In reviewing the history of obstetrics one is impressed by the agony and dangers to which women in labor were exposed, not only because there were no anesthetics or sedatives in use, but also because of the ignorance and barbaric practices of the well-intending but ill-informed midwives.

In the Middle Ages, a woman in labor was subjected to all manner of violence. She was entirely secondary to the child; the baby was all that mattered. The mother suffered such tortures as being tied by her limbs to a wooden bed while the attendants jumped upon her, lifted the bed and let it crash to the floor, or stood the bed on one end and bounced it to the ground, all in the hope of shaking the baby from its place. Until relatively recent times, only old men and women were in charge of labors.

Today the picture has changed completely. The mother is given foremost consideration. She is ready for labor mentally and her physical readiness is assured by the antepartum care she has received. She has the assurance today that little unforeseen can occur because she is in the hands of a scientist who has spent long years of preparation, by study and practice, in order to bring her safely through her ordeal and to crown it with the delivery of a fine healthy child.

The subject of labor can be discussed from any of several points of view for women approach it with varied and mixed emotions. Many women have a fear of the pains of labor; others think of their chances of not surviving or dread the thought of losing the baby. But the vast majority of women know full well that it is merely the termination of the pregnancy and either know what to expect or look forward to the time with great curiosity and hopeful anticipation. It is for the first groups that a few general assurances are given and for all expectant mothers that a scientific explanation of the expelled from the womb, through the vagina, into the outside world.

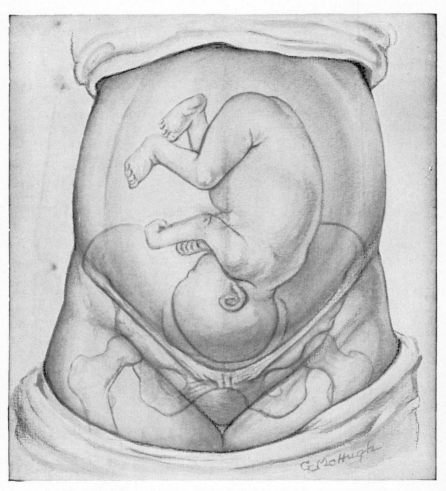

Fig. 20. Full term pregnancy with baby in normal position.

events accompanying this noblest of all womanly functions is presented.

Labor is the perfectly natural function by which the products of gestation, the baby and the afterbirth, are

THE ONSET OF LABOR

Labor Contractions. It is often difficult to decide when a patient actually is in labor, for frequently several weeks before term, or even

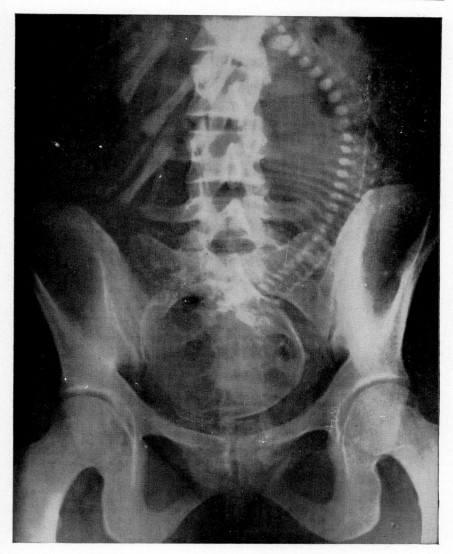

FIG. 21. X-ray corresponding to previous illustration.

at the time of the calculated date of confinement, the patient will notice regular painful uterine contractions which occur for a period of a few minutes to hours and then disappear, only to return in a similar manner or to develop into true labor contractions. These fruitless uterine movements are known as "false labor" and when entirely painless are called Braxton-Hicks contractions, or insensible labor.

True labor is characterized by rhythmical, painful uterine contractions, accompanied by typical changes in the lower portion of the body of the uterus and cervix. This definition cannot be applied to every case for, as in all phases of medicine, there are, inevitably, exceptions. Thus, a labor may terminate successfully without the contractions being either painful or regular. For practical purposes, when a patient has painful uterine contractions which occur at intervals of 5 to 15 minutes, or oftener, *and* last 30 seconds or longer, she is truly in labor. It is to be emphasized that the duration of the hardness of the uterus is no less important than the closeness of the contractions and that *both* factors must be present before one can be sure that real labor is present. Once these conditions are present the patient must now decide whether to call her doctor or to go to the hospital directly and let the hospital notify him that she has entered. It is presumed that the patient has visited her doctor many months before this time and that he has instructed her what his particular routine is. Some doctors wish to be called at any time and decide whether the patient should stay home a while or go immediately to the hospital; others prefer the patient to go directly to the hospital when they are sure that they are in labor during the night, but wish to be given notice during the day so their schedule can be revised accord-

ingly. If this subject has not been discussed already it should be taken up with the doctor in charge at the next opportunity. Naturally, if the patient awakens in strong labor or labor begins any time with frequent and strong contractions the doctor should be informed at once so that he can meet the patient at the hospital.

Labor rarely begins with the pains coming at regular intervals. Usually the patient gets a painful tenseness in her lower abdomen, back or rectum, followed by another contraction in 40 or 50 minutes. Gradually, these come at more frequent intervals and then there is no doubt about labor having begun. Often a patient will go to bed with no discomfort and awaken in active labor with only a five- to ten-minute interval between contractions. Occasionally a movie or bridge game will distract the patient so that she will not recognize labor until she retires. Then, in the quiet and stillness of the night, when every reaction is prominent or even exaggerated, comes the increased consciousness of any uterine contractions. This is partly responsible for the greater number of hospital admissions for labor at night, though no more babies are born at night than in the daytime.

Bloody Show. Often, about 24 hours before the labor begins, there is the passage from the vagina of a heavy mucus tinged or streaked with blood. It is often described as a pinkish or bloody mucous discharge. This is entirely normal and need cause no alarm. There is no need to notify your doctor when this occurs. It means that the cervix is undergoing changes characteristic of the beginning of labor, a "silent dilatation."

Bag of Waters. The bag of waters usually breaks with a gush after the patient has been in labor for some time and shortly before the delivery of the baby. Sometimes this fluid is lost hours or even days before the true onset of labor. In this case the doctor should be notified, for his conduct of the case will be determined in part by this information.

STAGES OF LABOR

For purposes of explanation and because each phase is distinct, labor is divided into three stages: first, the preparatory period; second, the birth of the baby; and third, the delivery of the afterbirth (or placenta).

First Stage. This lasts from the onset of labor until the baby is ready to be born. In primiparas, this takes usually about 14 hours, and in multiparas, about eight hours. The longer duration of labor in first confinements results from the fact that the passages are more tense and unyielding; when once dilated, a repetition is easier. Generally, the duration of labor, especially the first stage, also depends upon the strength and frequency of the labor contractions, the type of pelvis and soft tissues and the size and position of the fetus. The age of the patient has little to do with the duration and type of the labor. It is true that "old" primiparas (over 35) do have slightly longer labors and somewhat more often do present problems for the obstetrician, but not a difference sufficient to be a reason for worry for those involved.

When the various changes that take place in the body are understood, the discomforts are easier to

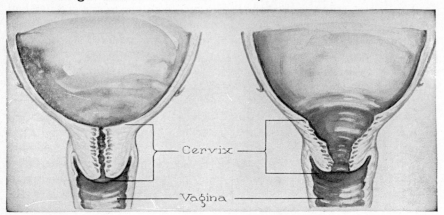

FIG. 22. The cervix at the end of pregnancy before labor begins (*left*) and the cervix opening and thinning during the first stage of labor.

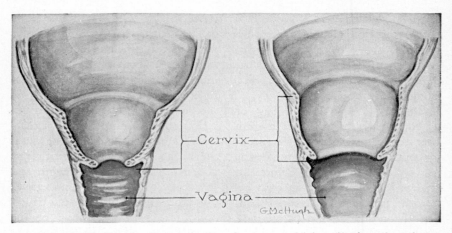

Fig. 23. The cervix during the late first stage of labor (*left*) and at the onset of the second stage of labor where it is completely dilated permitting the passage of baby through it.

bear. During this stage, some mothers become discouraged because no progress appears to be made. She may rest assured that every pain is for a purpose, and that results are being obtained even if she is not aware of them. The womb is a muscular organ which enlarges as the baby grows. It thus serves as an incubator, its initial purpose. When nature decides that the baby is to be separated from the mother, the womb loses its function as a carrier and becomes the chief contracting force which expels the baby from its cavity. The forces of this organ cause the lower portion of it, the cervix, to open up so that instead of the cervix being a narrow slit it becomes a wide, open passageway. When this occurs, the patient enters the second stage of labor.

Second Stage. As this is approached the bag of waters usually breaks, and the head descends deeper into the pelvis. The uterine contractions (labor pains) become more intense, and the patient has a bearing-down sensation. The perineum is stretched by the descending head, and the patient reflexly uses her abdominal muscles, straining as in having a bowel movement. In primiparas, about one to one and one half hours, and in multiparas, about 30 minutes are required to end this phase.

The vagina is capable of great distention at this time owing to the physiologic preparations by nature that took place during pregnancy. Nevertheless, almost invariably instruments (forceps) and an incision (episiotomy) are used in the delivery of the first baby, for this spares the mother many painful minutes and much effort, as well as preserving the good condition of the vagina, perineum and surrounding tissues.

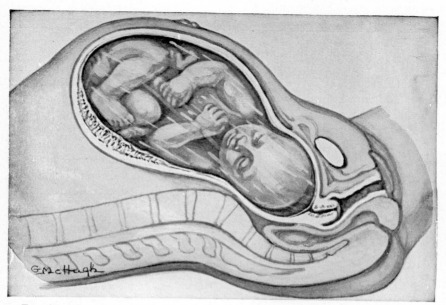

FIG. 24. The onset of labor with the bag of waters intact and the cervix undilated.

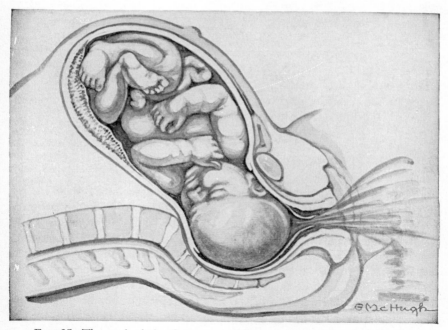

FIG. 25. The end of the first stage of labor with the cervix completely dilated and effaced. The baby's head has descended from the uterus into the lower passage. Note the breaking of the bag of waters.

Thus, a purposeful incision avoids a jagged tear which could involve important structures. The former heals better and with a much cleaner scar. Further, it saves the baby's head from being injured by the forces of labor pressing it against a resistant pelvic floor.

Third Stage. The placenta is closely attached to the uterine wall.

CONDUCT OF EARLY LABOR

Patient's Duties. When the patient suspects or knows that labor has begun she should call the doctor From this time on, nothing but light foods and fluids should be ingested. If a heavy meal has been eaten the doctor should be informed, as special precautions would then be necessary, particularly in the administration of

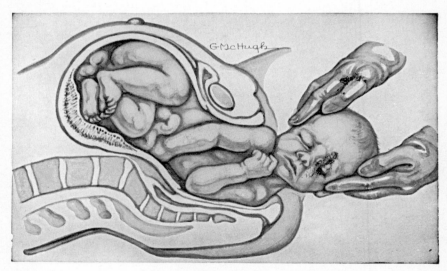

FIG. 26. The end of the second stage of labor.

It is a nonelastic structure which, even after the baby is born, does not shrink. After the baby is born the uterus, diminishing greatly in size, leaves little area for the placental attachment so it lies free in the hollow of the uterus. In five to fifteen minutes uterine contractions which are quite mild, expel it, completing the labor.

an anesthetic. Any recently acquired cough or cold, or any illness in the home, as scarlet fever, diphtheria or pneumonia, should be reported to the nurse or doctor upon admission to the hospital.

The husband may be present during most of the labor, but the delivery is a surgical procedure and is therefore one which visitors should not be permitted to witness. For this reason he is to leave the labor corridor during that time.

During the first stage of labor the patient should not bear down or "force," for any such effort is useless and exhausting. During the second stage, bearing down is encouraged; the doctor will decide when the time comes.

The mother should never touch her genitals while in labor, for germs from her nose or mouth or other sources can be transmitted thereby and be the cause of a serious infection.

If the bag of waters is not broken, the patient may assume any position comfortable for her, or walk about. On the other hand the doctor will decide whether she may be up or not if the bag of waters is not intact.

Nurse's Duties. After it is definitely established that labor is under way, the nurse carries out certain preliminary preparations for the delivery. These include shaving and washing with sterile soap the area over the pubic bone and about the orifice of the vagina. An enema usually is given, though under certain circumstances this is omitted. Then the patient is ready to be examined by the doctor or resident physician.

Doctor's Duties. An entrance history and check-up examination of the patient's general condition is made first, so that any recent or previously overlooked infection or defect is diagnosed and thus can be given the proper attention. This includes an examination of the heart and

lungs, the taking of the blood pressure and a urinalysis. Then an abdominal examination is made to determine the position of the baby, and the fetal heart tones are observed. Lastly, comes a rectal examination; for this method gives all the information about the progress of labor that is normally needed. This is a substitute for a vaginal or direct examination, which is omitted because of the danger of infecting the birth canal. Once in a while a vaginal examination is necessary because of uncertain rectal findings, in which case an elaborate cleansing preparation precedes.

The doctor need not stay with the patient during the entire first period. A resident physician or intern is only a few feet away to answer the patient's needs and make the necessary examinations. He will notify the doctor of her progress. The physician in charge will leave the orders for sedation, nourishment, fluids, etc., and examine the patient at regular intervals, so that he can be in attendance during the last part of the first stage and thereafter.

Unattended Delivery. Not rarely enough, though most unusually, a labor begins and terminates so rapidly that the baby delivers before the patient can be brought to the hospital or before a doctor can reach the patient—a so-called "precipitate delivery." Factors other than a very rapid labor may account for an unattended delivery. Among these are poor transportation, or failure on the part of the patient to recognize in

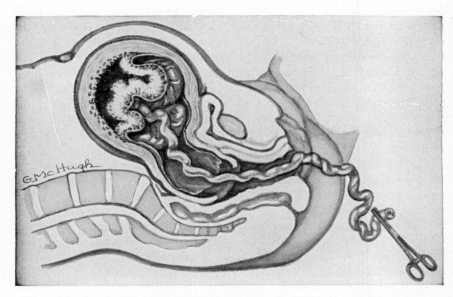

Fig. 27. The beginning of the third stage of labor, showing the uterus contracting and the placenta separating from it.

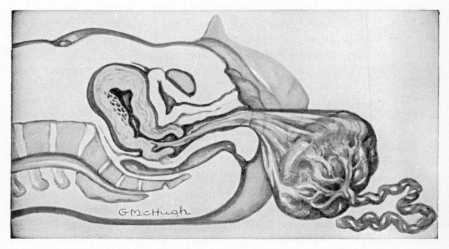

Fig. 28. The end of the third stage of labor. The uterus has contracted and the placenta has been expelled, pulling the membranes out with it. The uterus remains small and bleeding ceases.

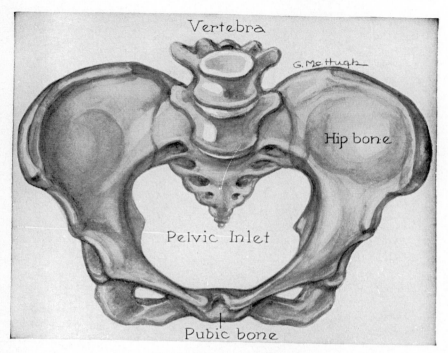

Fig. 29. The normal pelvis.

time the necessity to seek attention, seen especially among multiparas. When a precipitate delivery occurs the baby should be put in a protected place where it can breathe freely and be kept warm with blankets or towels. The mother also should be kept warm and comfortable. If the afterbirth and cord have been expelled from the uterus, they should be carried along with the baby. Nothing will happen if the cord is not cut, for nature has provided for the stopping of the circulation in the cord. When medical attention is found, the placenta will be inspected to see that it all has been released

from the uterus, the mother and baby will be examined for injury, and the necessary treatment will be given.

Dry Labor. Early breaking of the bag of waters—a day or so before labor begins—is attended by a so-called "dry" labor, the amniotic fluid having leaked out. This is, at times, the cause of a long labor or a complicated one, but in most instances in no way affects the outcome.

ANESTHESIA

Women have been taught to clamor for painless labors. Any technic or drug which is new and tends

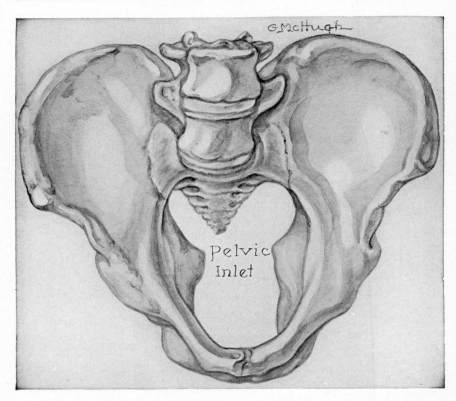

Fig. 30. A contracted pelvis. Note its asymmetry and narrowing of the inlet. Extreme contractions often necessitate cesarean section.

to relieve the pain of childbirth is given wide publicity, very often undeserved. *There is no drug which will cause the pain of labor to disappear completely and yet be perfectly safe for both the mother and the baby.*

There are two phases of relief of the pain of childbirth to be considered, the first and the second stages of labor.

During the first stage of labor some form of analgesic—a drug for the relief of pain—is routine. Another drug that produces amnesia (loss of memory) is selected, so that by this combination the patient has little pain and often only a faint recollection of that which was felt. The combination of morphine and scopolamine is commonly employed with excellent results. When repeated doses of scopolamine are given with one or more hypodermics of morphine, a desirable form of analgesia and amnesia is achieved, and is known as "twilight sleep." For best results the room should be darkened,

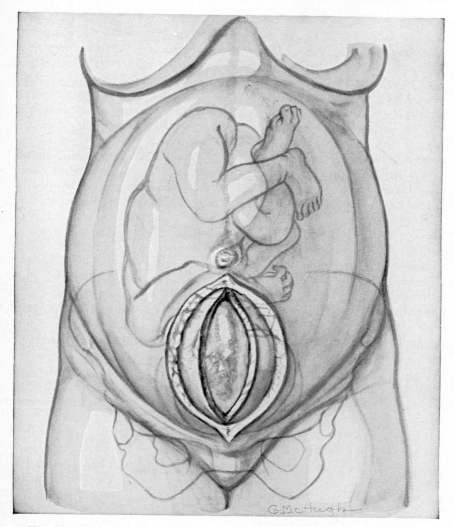

Fig. 31. Cesarean section. The incision is low in the abdomen and uterus; through this the baby is delivered.

and quiet must be maintained. In this state labor progresses, and the patient gets great relief from the uterine action, having little if any memory of the entire event. Used with caution in selected cases, this presents an excellent method of yielding relief. Other drugs can be substituted with equally good results. Complete anesthesia during the first stage of labor is possible only under certain special circumstances. Occasionally a patient has a painless labor with or without the use of drugs. At times, strong suggestions (a mild form of hypnosis) or hypnosis itself, can prove effective in eliminating pain. Lastly, caudal anesthesia or various types of spinal anesthesia may be used, though these are far from perfect. It can be said in their favor that in experienced hands and in selected cases they approach the ideal anesthetic.

There are several drugs which are available for the alleviation of the pains of labor and these will be used *to the fullest extend within the range of safety for both mother and baby.* The selection will depend, in part, upon the patient herself. Whereas one patient may find complete relief with a small amount of barbiturate or demerol or morphine, another patient may require heavy and repeated doses of certain sedatives. Besides the threshold of pain, there are other factors which influence the selection of the proper drug. For example, when a patient obviously is going to have a long labor a sedative must be chosen which has a prolonged effect, in contrast with the short-acting drug which is desirable for the patient who has borne many children before and is almost certain to have a rapid delivery.

The proper anesthetic for the second stage of labor depends upon many factors. The presence of tuberculosis or pneumonia precludes the use of a general anesthetic, so that some form of spinal or local anesthesia must be chosen or, if the former has been used during early labor, it serves for the termination of the second stage. A deep anesthetic is necessary for certain breech deliveries, and ether finds a good place here. Under average circumstances, ethylene or nitrous oxide provides a most suitable anesthetic for the birth of the baby.

Grantly Dick Read, an English obstetrician, has long been a pioneer in the movement to get women to look upon pregnancy and labor as perfectly normal and natural phenomena. Today several medical schools and many hospitals in the United States are teaching, with unquestionably excellent results, this so-called "natural childbirth." Actually it implies that early in her pregnancy the woman is put through a course of training which prepares her for her labor. This preparation ensures an adequate understanding of the anatomy and physiology of pregnancy and labor and includes exercises designed to strengthen certain muscles. The intimate relationship between body function and the mind is emphasized, and the patients are conditioned to the idea that labor can be painless if fear and apprehension are dispelled.

This method has many virtues and much can be said in its favor, yet, like so many other technics, it is not applicable to everyone. A woman who is curious about the method or desirous of having it should consult her physician and let him determine whether or not her particular case appears to be suitable for such

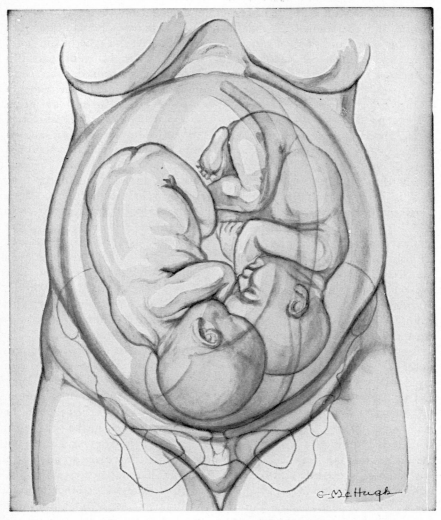

FIG. 32. Twin pregnancy. Each twin when born is usually smaller than a baby of a single pregnancy but the combined weight is greater.

a course of treatment.

By way of summarizing this subject, it may be said that the number of women who are enjoying practi-

cally painless labors is rapidly mounting. The physician prides himself in providing safe and sound relief. The expectant mother need no longer look to her impending labor with fear but rather with a feeling of confidence and the knowledge that it will be safe and not associated with undue pain or unpleasant memory.

Unusual Types of Births

Forceps Delivery. As was mentioned above, forceps are used arbitrarily in primiparas to effect an early delivery—the so-called elective, timely or prophylactic use of the forceps. In many deliveries their use is necessary because the uterine contractions and bearing-down of the mother are not sufficient to expel the baby, or because the baby's head has rotated in the wrong direction, and the application of the forceps is necessary to return it to the correct position. The forceps, originated by the ancients, developed by the Chamberlens and modified many times since, is an instrument which has saved many lives, both of mothers and of babies.

Cesarean Section. This is a major operation by which the baby is delivered through an incision in the abdominal and uterine walls. It is a common procedure and because it often spares the mother of all labor pains, patients occasionally request that it be done, unaware that it is not so safe for them or their babies as a natural delivery. When selected as the method of delivery, it is because there is present a condition, such as too-small pelvis or a tumor that blocks the passages, or other obstetrical complication that makes

vaginal delivery less safe than abdominal delivery. As a rule, a woman should have no more than three such operations. At the time of the third, her religion permitting, the patient is advised to be sterilized. This is accomplished by ligating the tubes, a procedure which in no way affects the sexual life of the woman.

Breech Delivery. When the doctor examines the patient's abdomen during the prenatal visits he will often find that instead of the head being low in the pelvis, the baby's breech (buttocks) lies there. At seven months this will be found more frequently than at term, for the babies more often than not turn spontaneously. An average of three in every 100 patients have breech babies when they go into labor. This type of delivery implies a slightly greater risk for the baby, but the mother's welfare is not jeopardized.

Abnormal Presentations. In about two out of 100 cases in labor the baby lies in an abnormal position in the pelvis, so that even though the head does descend in the pelvis first, it is deflected. The head may not come into the pelvis at all, but a shoulder descends first, as in a transverse presentation, or other unusual and unfavorable complications can occur, making the labor long and difficult and taxing to the utmost the strength of the patient and the skill and judgment of the doctor. Early recognition of the condition almost always ensures a favorable outcome, for at this time the management of these cases is not too difficult.

Multiple Birth. Twins are delivered about once in 89 pregnancies and triplets only once in some 7600 cases. The cause of multiple pregnancy is entirely unknown. There may be such a history on one side of the family, or on both sides, though this may be entirely lacking. In the event that a multiple pregnancy occurs, a repetition is quite likely.

The diagnosis of multiple pregnancy is verified by an accurate medical examination or x-ray evidence of two or more babies.

In two cases out of three, twins are of the same sex. This is readily understood for in this same proportion two eggs are fertilized by two spermatozoa instead of one egg by just one sperm. When the latter occurs, the egg divides to form identical twins, always of the same sex and possessing the same features and physical characteristics. Where two ova are involved in the development of twins, the chances are even as to whether the sex will be the same or not, and the likelihood of their resembling each other is no greater than in the case of any other sister and brother.

The babies in multiple pregnancies are usually born prematurely by two weeks, a fact which largely accounts for their small individual weight. Even when they go to term, each averages a pound less than a single fetus. Triplets weigh still less. However, their combined weight exceeds that of a single pregnancy.

10

Convalescence and After-Care

I feel that, in the heavens above,
The angels, whispering to one another,
Can find among their burning terms of love,
None so devotional as that of "Mother."
EDGAR ALLAN POE

In this world of ours nothing that is truly worth possessing is attained without persevering efforts and untiring vigilance. When a mother bends affectionately over her growing infant. the joy in her heart tells her that she is gazing on the most precious of all possessions. As the infant lies, appealing and helpless, dependent for all it has and is, a mother will feel that it was worth those special efforts to give it and herself proper nourishment during her pregnancy, to visit her doctor regularly and follow his instructions faithfully.

Now she must further take care of herself so that she can rear her infant well, providing him with the benefits of fresh air and sunshine, the comforts of cleanliness and appropriate clothes, guard him against disease and accident, and also direct with love and wisdom the first manifestations of a budding character.

The puerperium is the period after delivery which dates from the completion of the third stage of labor until six or eight weeks thereafter.

The obstetrician's duties do not end with the emptying of the uterus, but cover this entire period and include an examination at the end of it.

This time should be a most pleasant one for the mother. The long period of carrying the baby with all its discomforts is over, the abdomen is flat and she is able to move around freely and to enjoy her newborn baby. In order that the structures can return to normal more completely and quickly, certain rules pertaining to hygiene should be followed strictly.

PHYSIOLOGY OF THE PUERPERIUM

During the puerperium many physiologic changes take place in the maternal system, including alterations in metabolism, pulse and blood pressure. Waste products are excreted from the body and fluid is lost from the tissues, accounting for the large loss of weight in the early postpartum period. The womb shrinks down to normal size and casts off its protective lining. The vagina also undergoes certain regressive changes.

The breasts now well up and soon overflow with the nourishing fluid so important in giving the newborn an excellent beginning in life.

Within a few hours after delivery, patients often complain of a chill. This is due to absorption of by-products from the genital tract and is of no consequence. The pulse is very slow due to the change in blood volume and the lowering of the blood pressure. These return to normal in about ten days. The temperature is frequently slightly elevated at this time but in 12 to 24 hours it returns to normal and remains there.

Involution. Immediately following delivery of the baby and afterbirth, the uterus contracts into a hard mass which lies in the pelvis and lower abdomen with its upper border at the level of the navel. This is easily felt for several days, even in the patient who is quite obese. At this time it weighs about two pounds. Gradually it diminishes in size, a process that is noticeable from day to day, so that within ten days it no longer can be felt through the abdomen. By the end of six weeks the uterus is normal size, weighing now about two ounces. This process is known as involution and is brought about by a diminution in the size of each individual muscle cell. It is controlled partly by a relationship with the endocrine glands and accounts for the postpartum loss of a bloody fluid known as lochia. Involution is hastened when the mother nurses her baby. Occasion-

ally, she will be aware of the process by the occurrence of sharp cramps in her lower abdomen at this time.

Lochia. The lochia is formed of blood and the products from the breakdown of the lining of the uterus during the first week. At about the eighth day the lochia becomes pink instead of red, and two days later is yellowish; at the end of three weeks there should be no discharge whatsoever. The amount, as determined by the number of pads the patient will require, gradually diminishes. During the first week the patient will use about six pads a day and fewer thereafter. The odor closely resembles that of menstrual blood and can be controlled by the frequent changing of pads and the use of a deodorant. Occasionally the lochia will remain red for a period longer than two weeks, in which case the patient should notify her doctor, who will put her to bed and give medicines to aid involution. Conditions wherein the uterus has been greatly distended, as with twins or large babies, often account for a prolongation of the flow of bloody lochia.

Menstruation. The return of the menstrual flow is quite variable. Women who nurse their babies tend to have more of a delay than those who do not. Thus, in the nursing mother the menses usually returns in about two and one half months, and in those who do not nurse in about six weeks. The first period is very apt to be heavy, though again there is no consistency about this and it may be normal or even scanty. Furthermore, a few months may be required, once the flow has begun, for the regular cycle to be completely re-established. Some women will be a few days late during this time or even miss one or two periods. All the bleeding that may occur during this period is not necessarily the return of the menstrual flow. If it is prolonged or somewhat profuse, advice should be sought.

NURSING

Nursing at the breast is the best, easiest, simplest and most inexpensive way to feed a baby. Furthermore, the nursing mother does not have to worry about keeping her baby's milk free from harmful germs or from spoiling, nor does she have the fuss and bother of making the baby's feeding mixture, and of sterilizing bottles, nipples and other utensils.

Nursing a baby will not cause a mother to become fat, nor will it cause her breasts to become flabby, as is so often feared. A further advantage is that the baby's suckling is one of Nature's ways of helping to make the uterus, enlarged during pregnancy, shrink back to its normal size.

Nature intended that the baby should be fed at the mother's breast. That is why she put the food elements into breast milk in the right amounts for the young baby's needs. Furthermore, because breast milk forms small, finely divided curds in the stomach, it is the milk easiest for the baby to digest.

In addition to these important reasons, the milk in the breasts is always ready to be given. It is also fresh, clean and warm. It contains more iron than cow's milk, and the iron of mother's milk is absorbed and used about four or five times better than that of cow's milk. Some doctors believe that breast milk contains substances that protect the baby against disease. It is probable that the breast-fed baby has less chance of becoming sick than the bottle-fed baby and, if he is sick, has a much better chance of getting well.

Though breast feeding is enthusiastically advocated, the new mother should not feel depressed if she does not or cannot nurse her infant. The tenderness and the love that she demonstrates at all times, especially while feeding the baby, can compensate fully for the psychlogic advantages of breast feeding; the necessary vitamins and minerals can be added to an agreeable formula.

The Emotions and Nursing. The nervous condition of the mother should not be upset. Emotional states in the nursing mother can definitely affect adversely the quality of the milk she produces, causing severe stomach upsets in the infant besides affecting the quantity of milk secreted. Nursing, digestion and, in fact, all body functions are affected by the mind; cheerfulness has a favorable influence; depression, the reverse. The secretion of milk has been known suddenly to cease altogether under the influence of strong passion or deep sorrow, although this cessation is rare and never permament. Rather commonly, the quality and quantity of the milk is temporarily disturbed by the frets and worries of the mother, often due to anxiety over the baby, or over the nursing problem. Take success for granted, it is a more wholesome attitude.

It should be remembered that many drugs, condiments and alcohol appear in the milk. An occasional cocktail is harmless. Rich foods and anything that disagrees should be avoided selectively. Rest and recreation are important.

Onset of Lactation. The milk begins to flow usually about the third day, although in multiparas it may start a bit earlier and in primiparas a bit later. This onset of flow, when the "milk comes in," cannot cause fever; the assumption of "milk fever" has been disproved. Any rise in temperature at this time must be due to another cause; it will be investigated. The onset is often attended by hard, full and heavy breasts, which become tender and tense. This condition is called engorgement. Relief is usually obtained at once by nursing the baby and using a good nursing brassière or supporting binder between feedings. The condition is only temporary and usually lasts less than 48 hours, when the breasts become softer. Often sedatives are needed during the first few days until the baby is able to empty the breasts enough to give complete relief. This engorgement may require manual expression or the use of an electric breast pump, but this measure is best to avoid, for it tends to prolong the condition by stimulating the breasts to produce greater quantities of milk.

"Caking" is a condition of local engorgement, only one lobe or a few lobules being involved. This condition is transient and requires no active treatment.

Occasionally, mothers are startled by the appearance of a lump in one or both armpits. This is due to the existence of glandular tissue similar to that found in the breast. Such may become temporarily engorged or painful but soon recedes under the influence of pressure and ice packs.

The amount of milk secreted varies somewhat in the same mother and varies greatly in different mothers. The average amount secreted at first is about one half pint daily until the tenth day, when almost one pint is produced. By the end of the third or fourth week, this has doubled in many cases. There are other factors which influence the quantity and quality of the milk— the general condition of the mother, her physical make-up and, of course, the emotions, as already discussed. (See "Weaning," below.)

The baby is brought to the mother within eight to twelve hours after the delivery and put to the breast. This serves to stimulate the flow of milk. The first secretion is a milk-like substance called colostrum, which contains much that is nutritive. It is easily digested and serves as a laxative. The baby often will seem indifferent and listless, due to its new environment and the absence during the first two or three days of sufficient milk to satisfy its needs. If there is adequate glandular tissue and the nipples are everted, the baby soon learns how to nurse. A nurse will be on hand at this time to aid and instruct on how further to educate the newborn when this is necessary.

Time of Nursing. Following delivery the mother is given an eight- to ten-hour rest and a chance to recuperate and orient herself to her new status.

The baby is usually fed at regular intervals of four hours. A satisfactory and usual schedule begins at 6:00 A.M. with feedings at four-hour intervals thereafter. (Any beginning time is satisfactory provided the four-hour schedule is maintained.) Depending upon the conditions and sleeping habits of the baby, the 2:00 A.M. feeding (or corresponding early morning feeding if another time schedule is used) may be omitted. Some variation in the four-hour schedule may be necessary at first, until the milk comes in. Further, if the baby is small or weak, a three-hour schedule in the daytime and four-hour schedule at night may be advisable. Using the four-hour schedule, both breasts should be used for ten minutes each. Under the three-hour schedule, only one breast is used, and for a slightly longer period than ten minutes, at each feeding. Pediatricians vary somewhat in their ideas about the above discussion. The schedule best suited to the particular infant is the one selected.

The feeding of twins at the breast should not present any special difficulty, since the emptying of both breasts at every nursing seems to have a stimulating effect, and the mother is often able to nurse both babies without the addition of complementary food. Because they are usually small and lack resistance to infection, twins require much the same care as premature babies; they respond well to such careful management.

One twin is put to one breast, and the other to the opposite one for each feeding. They should be made to alternate from one breast to the other at every feeding, so that if one child nurses more vigorously than the other, both breasts will be stimulated equally. Twins should be put on a three-hour schedule until they weigh about 6½ pounds each when they can be changed to a four-hour routine.

Technic of Nursing. During the day, the daily bath should precede one feeding. The infant should never remain with the mother after nursing is completed, for the mother, falling asleep, could "overlie" and thus smother it.

Before each nursing the mother washes her hands and then carefully cleans her nipples, using merely soap and water.

The baby may have to be taught to

nurse at the breast for the first few times. Wet the nipple with breast secretion and while holding the baby's mouth on the nipple massage the breast toward it. If the nipple is retracted, endeavor to press the nipple and the areola (or brown area) into the baby's mouth. The sucking of the baby on the areola may help to bring the nipple forward. The continuous pulling of the nipple at each nursing will help to correct this retraction.

The most desirable position for the baby to be in as he nurses is a semi-reclining one, rather than a horizontal one, for he will take more milk and is less likely to swallow air, though the latter is almost unavoidable, regardless of the precautions taken against its occurence.

After each nursing it is a usual practice for the mother to "bubble" or "burp" the baby, i.e., the mother holds the baby over her shoulder and pats him gently on the back, thus releasing the bubbles of air. This makes the baby more comfortable and prevents the return of his food (bubble vomiting). This release of air from the stomach often stops babies from crying.

The nipples require no special care after the nursing period ends. They should be kept clean and dry, but no special solution or salve is necessary.

Nipple Shield. This is a round cup-shaped device composed of glass, plastic, or rubber material, which fits over the outer edge of the mother's nipple and has attached to

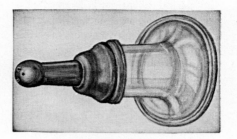

Fig. 33. Nipple shield.

it a rubber nipple for nursing. It is used to protect the nipples at the time of nursing when the nipples are inverted, cracked, or sore. Also, when the breast has to be pumped, the shield is useful. Breast feeding should be stopped if it is not possible to dispense with the nipple shield at the end of ten days.

Weaning. Transferring the infant's source of nourishment from the mother to the bottle. is often necessary. In the first place, the supply of the mother's milk may be entirely inadequate because of insufficient glandular tissue, inverted nipples, or a poor emotional reaction. Then again, the mother's physical condition may contraindicate nursing, as in tuberculosis or a breast infection. Other mothers may desire weaning so that they may go back to work; still others refuse to nurse for selfish reasons—the dread of developing large, pendulous breasts or of interference with their social activities. Whatever the reason, we now have methods for drying up the breasts rapidly and usually without much, if any, discomfort. After the period of nursing is over (this varies greatly, as the foregoing discussion and many other conditions would indicate), a tight binder should be applied to the breast. This ordinarily is sufficient, but if pain or engorgement occurs, ice packs and a mild analgesic, such as aspirin, should be used. There are drugs in the form of pills that some doctors prescribe. The results from their use are variable, and some physicians find them of little, if any, benefit. Many mothers, who have weaned their babies and have seen no milk or secretion for several days or weeks, will be startled to find that for no apparent cause there is a return of the milk after this time. This rarely is profuse and can be treated by re-applying a tight breast binder. Any discomfort that may exist can be managed as outlined above.

Wet Nursing. In some cases breast milk is essential to the life and well-being of the newborn. Formerly under these circumstances a wet nurse would substitute for the mother who was inadequate in this respect. Now, where breast milk is available in hospitals, or through bureaus and milk banks, and the care of the premature and feeble infant is much better understood, she is rarely employed. Some of the objections to wet nurses are the expense, the difficulty in finding a lactating woman at the proper time, and lastly the nuisance she can be; both she and the children she rears in this manner must be carefully ex-amined and also she must be available for the feedings at the proper times.

HYGIENE OF PUERPERIUM

Diet. The misconception that a pregnant woman must "eat for two" was discussed earlier, but this aphorism does apply to the nursing mother to a large extent, for the demands upon the mother for nourishment do not end with delivery; they merely assume another form and continue to increase as the infant grows.

After the first 24 hours, depending on the length and type of labor and anesthetic used, almost all patients are able to resume a regular diet. Inhalation anesthesia is often attended by nausea lasting 12 to 24 hours, but after that the appetite is usually good.

Throughout the entire nursing period the food should be such that it will provide adequate nourishment for the mother and aid in producing milk that will afford all that a growing, developing baby requires —food that will build a sound constitution. If the diet consists largely of meat, milk, eggs, fresh fruits and vegetables, supplemented by more tasty dishes, it will contain all the elements necessary to produce such milk.

The fluid intake must be adequate, the nursing mother needing at least two to three quarts daily, the non-nursing one less; 3000 calories is the daily requirements for the nursing mother, otherwise 1800, just as during pregnancy. A well-balanced diet, supplying all the materials needed by the nursing mother, must include each day the following foods:

1½ quarts of milk or substitute

1 egg or substitute

¼ pound of lean meat, fish or poultry (liver or kidney once a week)

½ cup of navy, kidney, lima or soybeans or peas or 2 tablespoonfuls of peanut butter or substitute

2 to 4 servings of vegetables

4 servings of fruit (2 citrus fruits daily)

1 serving of potato

6 slices of 100 per cent whole wheat bread or substitute

3 teaspoonfuls butter or enriched margarine

A sample menu is suggested as follows:

Breakfast
Orange juice

Poached egg Buttered toast

Wheat cereal

Milk

Coffee or tea as desired

Lunch
Old-fashioned navy bean soup

Stewed tomatoes

Fresh vegetable salad

Whole wheat bread Butter

Sliced peaches

Milk

Dinner
Meat loaf

Mashed potatoes Buttered spinach

Grapefruit and orange salad

Whole wheat bread Butter

Custard Milk

(Additional milk to be used between meals)

Weight. The mother loses considerable weight during the puerperium—from 12 to 15 pounds—returning to within a few pounds of her original status by the end of six weeks. This loss is greater in multiparas than in primiparas, in patients who went to term than in those who did not, in fat than in thin females. This loss of weight is due to the great activity of the organs of excretion and secretion—the skin, the kidneys, the bowels, the uterus and the breasts. Hence, nursing mothers lose more weight than the non-nursing.

Positions and Exercise. After the delivery and as soon as the patient is wide awake she is encouraged to lie on her abdomen for an hour and at least an hour twice daily thereafter. If she can sleep in this position it is even better. This aids in bringing the womb forward.

Also helpful for this purpose is the knee-chest position, which should be assumed for ten minutes in the morning, and again in the evening (Fig. 34). It is important that the knees be 12 to 16 inches apart, permitting air to enter the vagina. This should *not* be started until the baby is two weeks old! It should be continued until the baby is six weeks old, when the patient is examined.

Just as rest in the proper amount is necessary in the recuperative processes of the puerperium, so also is exercise. During pregnancy the muscles of the abdomen were under tension, were not in active use and thus lost much of their tone; the womb was far from its normal location, resulting in a stretching and twisting of its supports. Fat was deposited about the thighs, hips and abdomen. In order to accomplish a to derive the benefits intended. It is true that nothing can be accomplished in a few days and very little in a few weeks, but in several months the undesired fat pads will

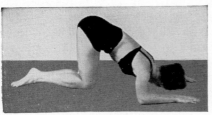

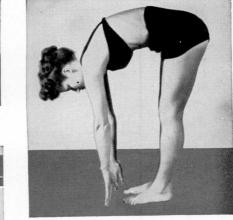

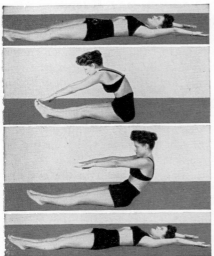

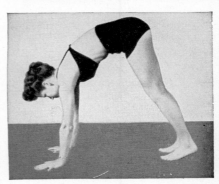

FIG. 34. Knee-chest position (*upper left*) and exercises designed to restore muscle tone after childbirth.

return to normal, certain exercises and positions are recommended.

It is quite important to remember to avoid fatigue, but a certain amount of persistence is necesary

have disappeared, and the dragging sensations in the pelvis often complained of will no longer be present.

A very important routine aids in the early return of the tone of the muscles of the perineum. The patient should lie flat on her back and raise her hips up off the bed a few inches. While in this position the muscles around the rectum should be contracted in the same manner by which a bowel movement is retarded. This exercise can be started on the third or fourth day. Later, the height to which the buttocks are raised can be increased and the perineum contracted more forcefully.

Cleanliness. Meticulous cleanliness is as important here as during the labor, for a patient may have a most difficult and successful labor, only to be infected during the recovery period. The perineum and vagina are to be treated as open wounds through which infection can gain access to the blood stream or into the deeper tissue. This is true regardless of whether there was an episiotomy done or a tear repaired or neither. The perineal pads are changed whenever they become soiled with lochia, and the genitals cleaned after each urination or defecation, as well as one or two additional times daily. As long as the patient does not have bathroom privileges, the nurse has this duty, in which case she places the patient on a bedpan and pours warm water over the vulva (pitcher douching), next using sterile cotton to dry, without rubbing, the area. The ambulatory patient performs for herself the same routine. Following urination the hygiene taught by the nurses is practiced and following a bowel movement the patient returns to her bed and receives care again from the nurse.

No vaginal douches are given, nor should the patient touch the vulva. Only when absolutely necessary is an internal examination done and this only with the strictest sterile technic.

As soon as the mother is able to walk she may take a sponge bath or shower. Tub baths must be delayed until the baby is three weeks old and douches until the baby is four weeks old.

Intercourse. Sexual relations must be avoided until the patient has been examined by her doctor when the baby has reached the age of six weeks.

The Bowels. If no evacuation has taken place, a mild laxative, selected by the physician, is given on the second day postpartum and an enema on the third day. Constipation is the rule for the first two or three weeks, but elimination improves steadily with the resumption of the patient's customary duties.

More careful attention given to the diet will also aid in establishing a daily regularity; eating bulky fruits and vegetables, drinking an abundance of water and attempting to have a bowel movement at the same time each day are all very important factors.

The patient who suffered the discomforts of hemorrhoids during pregnancy often has difficulty with them now. To gain relief, ice packs, rectal suppositories or a surface anesthetic will be prescribed. This condition rapidly improves, returning at least to a degree no more severe than it was before the pregnancy.

The Bladder. The bladder must always be emptied within the first ten or twelve hours after delivery and three times daily thereafter. Owing to the occasional compression of the neck of the bladder by the baby's head, the patient may find difficulty in urinating. Catheterizing (the insertion of a soft rubber tube) may be necessary, but other measures to induce voiding should be tried first. Placing a little steaming hot water in the bed pan, letting water run in the washstand, or gentle pressure on the bladder may suffice to stimulate the patient to urinate. The same causes that account for failure of urination also may explain the occasional incontinence (or involuntary loss of urine) experienced during the puerperium. This is only temporary, as a rule, and should cause no concern.

Sweating. As was mentioned under weight loss, part of this latter is due to the organs of excretion. The skin is no exception, and excessive perspiration, although especially noted in patients who have retained in their tissues undue amounts of fluid, is also found in the patient whose weight gain and fluid retention have been apparently normal. Keeping the patient dry is all that needs consideration.

POSTPARTUM PROBLEMS

Childbed Fever. In a small percentage of postpartum cases an infection develops somewhere in the generative canal; this is puerperal infection, sometimes called childbed fever. It can originate from a long labor, a tear during the delivery, from a pre-existing infection and not rarely from a cause or causes not apparent.

Now that it is realized that obstetrical cases require isolation and now that obstetrics itself has become largely a specialty in which doctors are trained to protect the mother from this and other latent dangers, childbed fever is no longer a threat to a woman's existence. Furthermore, the advent of sulfa drugs and penicillin, plus the wide availability of blood transfusions, has reduced the toll of this complication to a remarkably low level.

After-Pains. There are painful uterine contractions, menstruation-like cramps, which occur during the first few days of the puerperium. These are more troublesome to the multipara than to the primipara, there being greater muscle tone in the latter and hence the absence of large contractions. Nursing, itself, often initiates the contractions, reflexly on a hormonal basis, demonstrating the intimate connection between the uterus and the breasts and the central nervous system.

Depression. Regardless of how much the mother has longed for her baby, how easy her pregnancy and labor have been and the great delight shown by her husband and family, a large number of new mothers experience during the first two weeks postpartum one day of unexplainable mental depression. There seems to be little the doctor, nurse or family can do to alleviate this condition (descriptively called by some the "Baby Blues") but fortunately, within a period of about 24 hours, the patient returns to her former happy state and usually expresses amazement at having had this unpleasant though brief experience.

Stitches. There are many types of sutures that can be used in the repair of the vagina and surrounding passages. Sometimes sutures are used which require removal at the end of six or seven days while in other instances absorbable ones are employed. Just which type is chosen depends upon the length of labor, the size of the incision and other technical details. Occasionally, when absorbable sutures are used, a small piece of catgut (suture material) will work its way to the surface two or three weeks postpartum and give the patient undue concern. This is unimportant and leads to no complication.

Abdominal Binder. The idea that a binder will cause the abdominal muscles to return to their former strong condition has been abandoned. However, women who have a large, pendulous type of abdomen are often more comfortable with a tight binder.

Getting Up. Today following delivery early rising is generally advised. Instead of getting up on her eighth or ninth day, the patient is now allowed up on her second, third or fourth postpartum day for bathroom privileges. Shortly thereafter she can walk about at will. Just when the patient should walk depends largely on the type of delivery, her need for rest (more required if she has the care of a large family at home) and her recuperative powers, each case requiring individualization. Every precaution must be taken to preserve the patient's health and to prevent future disorders peculiar to the female. Adequate rest is essential.

Length of Hospital Stay. Following delivery the patient is to remain in the hospital eight to twelve days, an average of ten days. Due to overcrowding, especially during World War II and immediately after it, the hospital bed shortage was (and in some places still is) so acute that a hospital stay of only five to six days was possible. Ideally, a patient should remain under close observation for ten days, and longer if there was any complication.

Returning Home. Most patients are allowed to leave their homes after one week out of the hospital, but this again largely depends upon the course of the labor, the course and length of the hospital stay, the degree of responsibility with respect to housework and the care of other children which the patient has after her return home, and the number of flights of stairs to be traversed.

Visitors. During the puerperium the number of visitors is limited; this is for the mother's benefit. It reduces fatigue and eliminates the danger of infection being brought to the patient at a time when she is most susceptible.

Doctor's Visits. The doctor will see the new mother at least once daily during her hospital stay and more often if necessary. He will note from the record and his observations her progress and that of the baby, give instructions to the nurses regarding their care, and answer the questions which inevitably arise at this time.

Sixth-Week Checkup. A pelvic examination is not usually made during early convalescence, though at times this may become necessary. However, when the baby is six weeks old an examination is performed to determine the status of the external and internal genitalia, the patient's weight, blood pressure and general condition. Any abnormalities, such as a symptomatic displaced uterus or inflamed cervix, are corrected at this time or shortly thereafter. A very common condition involves the surface of the cervix and often accounts for leukorrhea, though it may not even cause this symptom. This is called a sore or blistering, technically known as an erosion. Although often discovered during pregnancy, it is usually not treated until the baby is from 2 to 3 months old.

Here a word about cancer prevention is in order, not to frighten the patient but to urge her to adopt a common-sense attitude about herself. In the concealed female organs minor or even serious conditions can

exist without causing pain, bleeding or other symptoms. Minor ailments can be treated promptly and thus will not develop into cancer. Even the latter, when diagnosed and treated early enough, rarely becomes dangerous. Hence, six-month examinations are advised for any woman who has had children or is beyond the age of 35. Such a plan causes little inconvenience or expense and gives the woman a sense of satisfaction and assurance that she is taking intelligent precautions.

Subsequent Pregnancies. How soon after a delivery should a woman become pregnant? Any time after 12 to 18 months. At this time the organs will have recovered completely from the changes and strain of the previous pregnancy, and the woman will be strong enough to undergo easily another pregnancy and labor. It is true an earlier conception would probably do no harm, provided the mother be given adequate relief at home from the burden of caring for her family and from other household duties.

Birth Control. In order to space offspring intelligently, parents must be familiar with a safe and well-understood method of avoiding the occurrence of conception. There are several methods that may be used with varying degrees of safety. In the choice of a particular method much depends upon the patient's religious and moral views. Also important is the patient's ability to grasp the use of a complex method and of equal significance is her anatomic structure, certain abnormalities precluding the use of various mechanical means.

For those who wish to avoid the use of artificial means, there are two methods of relative safety. (1) The "safe period" is based upon the rhythmic regularity of the menstrual cycle. Most women ovulate 14 days before arising and before any food or fluid is swallowed. The day before the egg is released from the ovary there is a slight drop in temperature and the next day near the time of ovulation there is marked rise, as much as eight-tenths of a degree or even a full degree. Intercourse is avoided from the time of

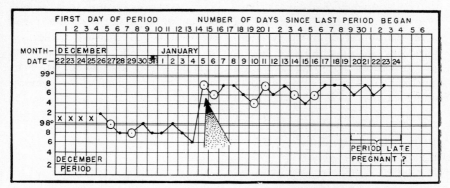

FIG. 35. Typical basal temperature curve. Arrow points to the day when temperature rises sharply. This is the approximate ovulation time and the peak of fertility.

before the onset of their period. In fact, some can actually state the exact time, for they are conscious of a sharp pain in the left or right lower quadrant, the so-called "mittelschmerz" or intermenstrual pain. In order to apply this knowledge practically, total abstinence is maintained for a period of five days before ovulation and five days after ovulation. (2) The Roman Catholic Church now permits the application of our knowledge of the time of ovulation based on the basal temperature curve. Figure 35 illustrates a typical curve during a menstrual cycle. The oral temperature is taken each morning the premonitory dip until three days after the marked rise. When followed carefully, these methods are reasonably satisfactory. Failures occur when the schedules are not calculated carefully or when ovulation occurs at an exceptional time during the cycle. Because the second method usually detects this, it is more effective.

It is possible also to determine the time of ovulation by studying slides made from the mucous secretion of the vagina—the so-called "vaginal smear" method. This technic can be employed in conjunction with the basal temperature curve, but before it can be solely relied upon, it will be necessary to conduct further investigation in this field.

By far the most accurate method of predicting the time of ovulation is by the rat test. A small amount of the subject's urine is injected into a young female rat. About four hours later the ovaries of the rat are examined, and when ovulation is about to occur in the patient the ovaries of the rat appear quite red with engorged blood. Since this is a laboratory procedure requiring skill and experience it is most widely used in aiding couples with low fertility to conceive rather than in the prevention of conception.

For those who wish to learn of the mechanical means of birth control, it is suggested that advice be sought of the obstetrician. He will select the appropriate method and explain the best way to employ it.

There is another method which deserves mention because it is widely, if not wisely, used. In coitus interruptus the male partner withdraws before completion of the sexual act. It is not a safe method and is undesirable for psychological and physiologic reasons.

11

The Newborn

"What am I?
An infant crying in the night;
An infant crying for the light;
And with no language but a cry."
TENNYSON

At birth the baby undergoes a distinct change of environment. He is no longer a completely protected tenant but a physiologically independent being, capable of respiring, excreting and growing.

As a rule the baby begins to breathe and cry within a few seconds to minutes after birth. He has an immediate demand for oxygen because the placental circulation at this time is no longer functioning. His respiratory center is stimulated by the impure blood which accumulates in the uterus due to the lack of oxygen, and by contact with air, which is at a lower temperature than that of the uterus. His color soon changes from a dusky blue or pale pink to a healthy rosy one.

Where heavy sedation or a long anesthetic has been administered, as with a difficult birth, the baby may not breathe for as long as eight to ten minutes, and then the attendant often has to stimulate him in one or several ways, determined by the individual case.

This sudden separation at birth from the placenta means much more than just a loss of oxygen to the newborn. Within the child changes must take place which affect every system in the body—respiratory, circulatory and excretory. The organs which have been present though inactive for so many months are suddenly called into use. The lungs expand, blood is diverted into new channels, and the kidneys perform. This metamorphosis is quite complex and when it is studied, one is as amazed at this phase of life as at the miracle of conception itself.

Knowledge about the newborn means freedom from worry. The mother who is going to assume the chief care of her infant should know what is normal and abnormal and be able to recognize these conditions in her baby. Some hospitals have classes for mothers, where demonstrations are given on how to care for and bathe the newborn. Instruction in child care can also be obtained from appropriate and authoritative books and from the attending pediatrician.

It is advisable that the newborn be placed in the care of a doctor (preferably a pediatrician) as soon as possible after birth, regardless of his condition. Most pediatricians want

THE NORMAL NEWBORN INFANT

Identification. Babies are identified so accurately and completely that a mixup is impossible. As soon as the baby is born and the cord is tied, a number is secured to the stump of the cord, and an adhesive

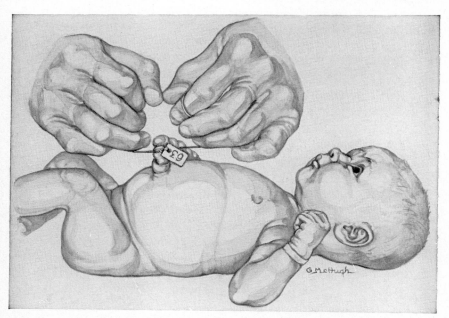

FIG. 36. Treatment of the umbilical cord. This is ligated and cut about one inch from the abdominal wall. A special tie is used and has a number attached.

to see the baby soon after birth and before he leaves the hospital, about once each month after this during the first year, and at less frequent intervals thereafter.

With this introduction, it is now in order to describe the average normal infant, how he looks and behaves at birth and during the first few days of his existence.

strip with a number on it is placed on the baby's back. A numbered band is also placed around the wrist. These three numbers are entered on the mother's hospital record and correspond to a number placed about the mother's wrist. Also, the baby's palm and/or sole prints are placed with the record. These methods, and various other ingenious ways of identification that hospitals employ, such as the use of beads spelling the mother's surname and placed about the baby's neck or wrist, should leave no doubt in the mother's mind that the baby she holds is her own.

Weight. There is a wide normal variation in the weights of full-term babies, ranging from five to eleven pounds at birth. First babies are gen-

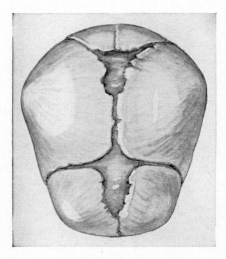

FIG. 37. Skull of the newborn.

erally smaller than succeeding ones. The baby weighing only five pounds may be just as healthy as the heavier ones. If the birth weight is under five pounds the infant is regarded as a premature or immature infant, depending upon whether or not the pregnancy was carried to full term. Boys generally weigh about three ounces more than girls, and the average for the former is just under seven and one half pounds. The smallest baby known to survive

weighed about one and a half pounds, the largest on record, 25 pounds. During the first three to five days there is a weight loss averaging about seven to eight per cent of the birth weight, a perfectly normal anticipated phenomenon. This is because the newborn takes little nourishment during this period, and loses fluid by way of the kidneys, bowels and skin. At the end of ten days to two weeks the baby usually weighs the same as when born. A baby normally gains from five to eight ounces weekly during the first six months of life.

Height. The average height, or crown-to-heel measurement at birth is 20.5 inches for full-term infants, males being a fraction of an inch taller than females.

Head. The average circumference of the head at birth is 13.9 inches for males, and 13.5 inches for females.

Usually, in all but very rapid labors, the head is molded as the baby moves through the birth canal, and the changes which result are often a cause of undue worry for the mother. One of these changes is a soft lump on the side of the head called a caput succedaneum. It is temporary and will completely disappear by absorption in from seven to ten days. When forceps are used, an impression of the blades of this instrument may be left on the cheeks. It is of no consequence and fades altogether in several days.

The skull of the newborn is made up of several variable-sized bones. Where they fail to meet completely, as on the front and back of the head, two soft spots result. These are known as the anterior and posterior fontanelles respectively. The posterior or smaller fontanelle usually closes up within six to eight weeks after birth, whereas the larger one

Nails. The finger and toe nails are well developed at birth. They grow rapidly and have to be cut at frequent intervals to prevent the baby from scratching himself.

Teeth. Rarely a baby is born with one or several teeth. This is quite

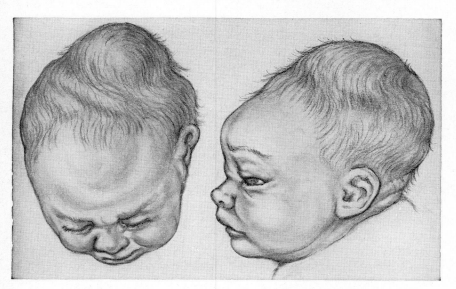

Fig. 38. Molding of baby's head by its passage through the birth canal. This is a frequent occurrence and one soon remedied by growth.

closes by the 15th or 18th month of life.

Chest. The chest of the newborn infant measures one half inch smaller in circumference than the circumference of the head.

Hair. At birth there is a variable amount of fine, soft, dark hair, which falls out in part near the second week of life. Gradually new hair grows in, of firmer texture and usually lighter in color.

unusual, since the average infant does not usually cut teeth until the sixth or seventh month when the two lower central incisors appear.

Bowels. During the first few days of life the stools consist of a dark green, tarry material called meconium, which is a waste product formed in the child's intestines during the last months of pregnancy. Soon the color of the bowel movement becomes lighter and normal stools appear. These, in the case of breast-fed babies, are bright yellow in color and of a smooth, pasty consistency. One to four bowel movements daily is the rule during the first month of life, but breast-fed babies may have only one in two or three days and remain well. It is the consistency which is important.

Urination. The first urine usually appears 12 to 36 hours after birth, although it often occurs at birth. The urine is highly acid. Suspension of urination for the first 24 hours need cause no alarm if the infant is otherwise normal. When it persists, it may be due to some malformation in the genito-urinary tract, which can be readily detected.

Hearing. Infants are deaf for the first 24 hours after birth. This condition sometimes persists for two or three days, after which the hearing gradually develops and becomes very acute during the early months of life.

Touch. The tactile sense is present at birth but is not generally well developed except in the lips and tongue, an obvious prerequisite for proper nursing.

Taste. This is highly developed at birth. Sweet and sour can be distinguished and a slight variation in the formula is occasionally sufficient cause for the newborn to accept or refuse the bottle. Sweet substances excite the sucking movements and are always easily administered.

Smell. The results of experiments are inconclusive concerning the development of this special sense in the newborn, though it is probably present to some extent in all newborn infants and especially well developed in those infants born blind. This ability reaches its peak of development much later than the other senses.

Mouth. The doctor removes all the mucus, blood and amniotic fluid from the baby's throat and mouth at birth so that he will not suck these into his lungs, and also to assist him to breathe freely. Other than gently swabbing out the mouth with gauze and weak boric acid solution at birth, further swabbing and washing is forbidden to prevent infections such as thrush.

Tongue tie is relatively common but usually requires no cutting unless the tongue cannot be protruded beyond the lips, or the tie prevents the infant from eating.

Sleep. Babies sleep almost continuously for the first two or three days. Thereafter they usually spend 20 of the 24 hours in slumber.

Navel. The umbilical cord is tied or clamped, and cut, immediately after birth. The stump is treated with an antiseptic and a dressing and binder are applied. The cord generally dries up and separates at the end of the first week, though at times it may normally remain attached a little longer. If, after falling off, moisture or drainage exists, an alcohol dressing or a drying powder should be applied to the navel. In some instances after the cord has fallen off, dark red granulation tissue (so-called "proud flesh") may remain. This usually requires cauterization by a physician.

Due to moderate weakness and separation of the abdominal muscles, the navel sometimes bulges. This is not due, as some believe, to neglect on the part of the attending physician. Treatment of this bulging, called hernia, depends upon its size. Usually all that is necessary is to bind and hold the muscles together by a strip of properly placed adhesive plaster.

Eyes. A fresh solution of one per cent silver nitrate is put into each eye to prevent infection and possible blindness. This is done shortly after the baby is born, at the time the umbilical cord is tied.

At birth the eyes are usually a pale blue color. The color may change at any time within the first year of life. The eyelashes and eyebrows are very short and fine, and barely visible. The baby is able to react to light at birth, closing his eyes in the presence of a bright light. The pupils can be seen to contract at such a time. Actual ability to see and distinguish objects develops rapidly within a few months. The muscles of the eyes act irregularly, failing to co-ordinate, but by the end of the first four to six months co-ordination is attained. Usually by the end of the first month, though at times somewhat later, tears flow when the baby cries. The presence of tears helps wash away any irritating particles in the infant's eyes.

Skin. The usual color of the baby is a pink to deep red at birth. The majority of babies develop a varying degree of jaundice a few days after birth. This condition usually disappears by the end of the first week. It seldom needs any treatment. It is common to see tiny, scarcely visible, white spots on the face, especially about the nose. These are due to closed, inactive sweat glands and disappear in about a month when the glands begin to function. The soft down hair often seen on the surface of the baby usually is gone by the end of the first week of life. The more common birthmarks are brown or black moles, and pink-to-red areas on the skin known as blood spots, or angiomas. The latter are due to a dilation of tiny blood vessels of the skin. Moles and angiomas rarely disappear. Some tend to fade, others require treatment.

Temperament. It is unwise to generalize about controversial subjects such as the effects of heredity versus environment, but the old saying, "Like father like son," can be applied to the newborn, and we feel that another axiom is appropriate, "Like mother like child." Rather consistently one finds fewer colicky, irritable, difficult babies among stable, emotionally well-balanced mothers than in the opposite worrisome group. The only benefit that can be derived from such a brief statement as this is to create an *awareness* of this possible influence, such being the first step in making progress toward a healthier attitude not only toward the raising of children but toward life itself.

UNUSUAL CONDITIONS OF
THE NEWBORN

Considering the difficult journey made by the infant as he travels through the birth canal and the many changes which he must undergo immediately after birth, it is little wonder that some infants have a bit of difficulty at first in making the necessary adjustments. The expectant mother may have heard about the unusual conditions which can occur in newborn babies. Due to frequent exaggeration, which often causes mothers undue worry, some of the commoner conditions will be briefly dealt with, leaving the more detailed matters to the pediatrician.

Menstruation. Correctly called pseudo or false menstruation, this condition occurs in about five per cent of newborn baby girls. It consists of a slight show of blood from the vagina, occurring on a glandular basis, just as swelling of the breasts in the newborn. Lasting, as it usually does, only a few days, this condition is of no consequence.

Breasts. Babies of both sexes often exhibit swelling and engorgement of the breasts. Occasionally a water secretion is seen exuding from the nipples. This is caused by the same hormone which stimulates the mother's breasts. Since the intimate relationship between mother and baby ceases to exist at birth, this hormone soon disappears from the baby's blood and in a week the breasts become normal. The treatment is to leave them alone; manipulation or massaging can only result in harm.

Dehydration Fever. There is a normal loss of body fluid after birth due to respiration, bowel movements and urination. If this loss continues and exceeds the infant's intake of fluids, the baby may suffer from dehydration. The infant's temperature may rise, the skin becomes dry, the fontanelles sink, and there is a further loss of weight. The administration of sufficient fluids during the first few days, together with an adequate milk intake afterward, usually prevents progress of this condition and it is soon overcome without further difficulty.

Malformations. This could be an alarming subject, but when parents realize the extreme rarity of such conditions their minds should be at ease. The subject is discussed only for the sake of completeness. The presence of congenital malformations of the external organs, such as harelip, is obvious enough. When the internal organs are involved the resultant symptoms usually aid the physician in reaching an early diagnosis and plan of treatment. Most conditions are compatible with life, though rarely a baby is born with organs so ill formed that he is unable to survive.

Sometimes a baby is born with an abnormality of the heart, so that mechanically its action is imperfect and he is unlikely to survive. When this situation exists, the circulation throughout the entire body is inadequate and any exercise or exertion by the baby leads to a cyanotic color of the body. These are known as "blue babies."

Birth Injuries. What has been said of malformations applies to some extent to birth injuries. The latter are relatively rare but of them many, unfortunately, occur in simple spontaneous deliveries as well as in the difficult ones. Naturally, they are more common in difficult deliveries. Among them are injuries to the brain or spinal cord, resulting usually in hemorrhage. Fractures of the extremities, skull or clavicle, and dislocations of any of the joints may occur. The latter two types of injuries, when recognized early and properly treated, heal readily and are rarely serious.

Erythroblastosis (blood disease of fetus and newborn). A certain small percentage of babies die within the mother's womb several weeks before birth, or shortly thereafter. Some of these babies are diagnosed as having erythroblastosis, a disease given much publicity of late with the discovery that its cause is an incompatibility between the Rh blood factor in the mother and father. The occurrence of any such disturbance in a baby because of Rh differences in the parents is not frequent enough to give prospective parents any concern. Examination for the Rh type is routine and should an incompatibility exist the various possibilities will be discussed with the parents.

SPECIAL CONSIDERATIONS

Circumcision. Some doctors maintain every boy should be circumcised at birth for purposes of cleanliness.

Certainly it is a fact that washing of the genitals is much easier if this has been done, otherwise the foreskin must be retracted at each bath to maintain adequate hygiene. While most boy babies may not require circumcision, a long and tight foreskin which cannot be easily pushed back after several attempts requires excision. This is a simple operation, done any time from the fifth to the ninth day. The aftercare consists merely of applying petroleum jelly dressings to the penis, and avoiding irritation and uncleanliness to the newly operated area.

Premature Infants. A premature birth is one that occurs at the seventh month or at any time thereafter before term, regardless of the infant's birth weight. An immature baby is one which is born at term but weighs less than five pounds. Both types require special care and supervision, since they are prematurely or immaturely developed. The best incubator by far is the uterus. The closer to term the baby is when born, the better developed he will be and the greater his chances of survival will be. To repeat an earlier statement there is absolutely no truth in the idea that a baby born at eight months has less chance of living than one born at seven months. The premature infant's powers of resistance are less, his respiratory, digestive and circulatory systems are relatively feebly developed, and the muscles are quite weak. Thus his needs for expert care are much greater. The innovation of modern incubators and our greater knowledge of just what these small babies require in the way of nursing care, plus the advent of new bactericidal drugs, have made the outlook for these small babies a bright one indeed.

SUMMARY OF CARE OF THE NEWBORN

The actual guidance for the care of the newborn is left entirely to the pediatrician; however, a summary of the underlying principles for the development of a healthy baby are here in order and will serve as food for thought for the mother. These principles are:

1. Proper food
2. Sunshine and fresh air
3. Rest and sleep in proper amounts
4. Cleanliness of clothes, food and surroundings
5. Regularity in daily routine
6. Frequent consultation with the baby's doctor

BIRTH CERTIFICATE

The birth certificate is filled out completely and signed by the physician before the patient leaves the hospital. The name chosen for the baby is given to the nurse. It is wise for the parents to decide on two names before the patient goes to the hospital. The certificate is mailed to the Board of Health, Department of Vital Statistics. Should you desire a photostatic copy, such can be obtained by mailing one dollar to this bureau at the City Hall in your city.

LAYETTE, NURSERY AND
NURSERY NEEDS

Most large department and infant-wear stores have layette and nursery supplies listed but such outlines are often incomplete or confusing to the mother, especially to the "new" mother. Therefore, a complete description of the layette essentials, the needs for a nursery, the bath essentials and also the feeding and sleeping equipment that is desirable are now presented.

Layette. There are only a few considerations to keep in mind when selecting a basic layette for the newborn. First and foremost is the comfort and health of the child. Although cotton knit binders, shirts, gowns and kimonos are the choice of the largest number of doctors, this may be modified to part wool garments where the climate is "rugged" in winter, and where the heating is inadequate or because of the doctor's personal preference. A 10 per cent wool content is sufficient to add warmth, absorb moisture and yet not irritate the baby's sensitive skin. The opinion is rather general to have cotton next to the baby's skin and add warmth when necessary by using wool sacques, sweaters, blankets, etc., outside.

Experiment has proved that infant's undergarments, when made of fine-combed cotton yarn, will keep their shape because of the elasticity in the weave which is permanent. Such garments are more comfortable even after frequent washings. A good quality cotton garment absorbs moisture much like a blotter, washes easily, can be boiled when necessary and dries quickly; thus requiring no extra work for the mother.

DEPARTMENT OF COMMERCE BUREAU OF THE CENSUS	STANDARD CERTIFICATE OF LIVE BIRTH	State File No. .... Registrar's No. ....

State of ....

1. PLACE OF BIRTH:	2. USUAL RESIDENCE OF MOTHER:
(a) County	(a) State ....
(b) City or town .... (If outside city or town limits write RURAL)	(b) County ....
(c) Name of hospital or institution:	(c) City or town .... (If outside city or town limits write RURAL)
.... (If not in hospital or institution give street number or location) (d) Mother's stay before delivery:	
In hospital or institution .... In this community .... (Specify whether years, months, or days)	(d) Street No. .... (If rural give location)

3. Full name of child	4. Date of birth .... (Month) (Day) (Year)

5. Sex:	6. Twin or	If so—born 1st,	7. Number months of
....	triplet	2d, or 3d	pregnancy	8. Is mother married? ....

FATHER OF CHILD	MOTHER OF CHILD
9. Full name...	15. Full maiden name ....
10. Color or race .... 11. Age at time of this birth......yrs.	16. Color or race .... 17. Age at time of this birth .... yrs.
12. Birthplace .... (City, town, or county) (State or foreign country)	18. Birthplace .... (City, town, or county) (State or foreign country)
13. Usual occupation	19. Usual occupation ....
14. Industry or business	20. Industry or business ....
21. Children born to this mother:	22. Mother's mailing address for registration notice:
(a) How many other children of this mother are now living?	....
(b) How many other children were born alive but are now dead?	....
(c) How many children were born dead?	....

23. I hereby certify that I attended the birth of this child who was born alive at the hour of .... m. on the date above stated and that the information
given was furnished by ...., related to this child as ....
24. Date received by local registrar	Attendant's own signature ....
25. Registrar's own signature	M. D., midwife, or other .... Date signed ......
26. Date on which given name added .... by .... Registrar	Address ....

UNITED STATES STANDARD CERTIFICATE OF BIRTH

Why births should be registered.—There is hardly a relation of life—social, legal, or economic—in which the evidence furnished by an accurate registration of births may not prove to be of the greatest value, not only to the individual, but also to the public at large. It is not only an act of civilization to register birth certificates but good business, for they are frequently used in many practical ways, some of which are listed below:

(1) As evidence to prove the age and legitimacy of heirs;

(2) As proof of age to determine the validity of a contract entered into by an alleged minor;

(3) As evidence to establish age and proof of citizenship and descent in order to vote;

(4) As evidence to establish the right of admission to the professions and to many public offices;

(5) As evidence of legal age to marry;

(6) As evidence to prove the claims of widows and orphans under the widows' and orphans' pension law;

(7) As evidence to determine the liability of parents for the debts of a minor;

(8) As evidence in the administration of estates, the settlement of insurance and pensions;

(9) As evidence to prove the irresponsibility of children under legal age for crime and misdemeanor, and various other matters in the criminal code;

(10) As evidence in the enforcement of law relating to education and to child labor;

(11) As evidence to determine the relations of guardians and wards;

(12) As proof of citizenship in order to obtain a passport;

(13) As evidence in the claim for exemption from or the right to jury and military service.

Fig. 39. Birth certificate.

If the baby's laundry is to be done at home, a minimum number of each item will be sufficient provided the clothing is washed daily. If the commercial laundry is to be used, a much larger number of each garment will be required to tide over from one delivery to the next.

The size is an important consideration when selecting the layette. A garment too small will bind and restrict, a garment too large will wrinkle and bunch up under the child. The first size, usually known as "infant size," is preferable for the newborn.

In selecting diapers, gauze is preferred because it absorbs quickly, washes easily and dries quickly. Flannel is the last choice because the material absorbs so slowly, the urine runs off before it is absorbed and the baby gets very wet and cold. Cotton knit diapers are very good for night use as the material helps to keep the body's warmth in; but it dries so slowly that it is unwise for 24-hour use unless there is plenty of drying space.

Disposable diapers (moisture repellent pants and disposable pads) are a great help to the mother who does not have help when she first returns from the hospital with her baby, or when traveling.

Dresses of various materials, within a wide price range, may be obtained at all department stores, or if preferred, patterns may be purchased and the dresses may be made. The gertrudes (slips), depending on the season, may be of flannelette, cotton knit and nainsook. It is not wise to put wool or silk next to the skin. The wool may irritate the tender skin while the silk feels cold.

Most pediatricians recommend that the baby's feet be kept bare while they are in bed and for a short period each day for exercise. Short booties may be put on when the child is picked up, and on special occasions for warmth. Long stockings or booties can be worn at night if weather is extremely cold and the heating inadequate. Long-sleeve shirts and long stockings under the nightgown will give added protection and warmth so that fewer blankets will be needed and the baby will have freedom to kick and stretch and pull.

ESSENTIALS

Abdominal binders (bands or belly bands) 4 to 6 (form-fit preferred) Not all pediatricians feel that these are desirable or useful: the decision for their use should be left with the attending physician

Sleeveless shirts (pinning bands) 4 to 6

Elbow length Jiffon or tie shirts 4 to 6

Long sleeve Jiffon or tie shirts 4 to 6 (if weather is cold and rugged)

Nightgowns (cotton knit, flannelette or outing flannel) 3 to 4

Kimonos (cotton knit, flannelette, outing flannel, spun rayon or seersucker) 3 to 4

Diapers 4 to 5 dozen (preferably gauze 20 x 40)

Disposable diapers (4 pants and 4 boxes of 48 to start) disposable pads

Moisture-proof panty (so-called rubber panty) 1 only for social security for person holding baby. For use only when going out

Wool soaker (panty or trunk) very desirable to put over diaper. Absorbs moisture, keeps body warmth in, yet permits air to circulate

Safety pins, 1 card large or medium, 1 card small size

OPTIONAL (Sometimes received as gifts)

Dresses and gertrudes (slips) usually selected together of similar material

Kimono and gertrude (slip) sets of either flannelette or cotton knit

Bunting (if Fall or Winter baby)

Coat and bonnet of silk or fine wool for dress or christening

Shawl (hand woven, usually wool or wool and silk thread) for all seasons

Sacques, bonnet or cap and bootie sets

Baby's Nursery. The baby's nursery should be sunny and well ventilated. If sunny it is less humid and there is less organic matter. The temperature should not be over 70° in the day and not more than 65° at night for the first two months. Later, a greater extreme is allowed. Have good ventilation without draft.

Sleeping equipment (see below)

Linoleum or throw rugs

Chest of drawers

Scale

Waste receptacle

Screen to prevent draft

Chair (low, for mother)

Hamper

Dressing table (bathinette serves very well)

Baby's Tray. This should be conveniently located, either in the baby's room or in the bathroom. It contains all the items for the baby's proper hygiene.

Soap, oil and powder manufactured only for baby use

Absorbent cotton

Jar set (sterile water, boric acid solution, cotton pledgets, oil, etc.)

Wash cloths

Towels (small absorbent for face and head, large absorbent for bath)

Bath apron, bath spray

Bath thermometer

Bath tub or bathinette. The latter is preferred if income and space permit. It is invaluable for bathing, dressing and changing the baby, to say nothing of saving the mother's back and energy.

Laundry Equipment

Diaper pail

Water softener if necessary

Soap (mild nonalkali)

Washer if desired

Clothes rack or reel for drying

Clothes line and clothes pins

Feeding Equipment

Nursing units (complete with nipple, cap, etc.) 6 8-oz. and 2 4-oz. bottles if baby is formula fed every four hours. More will be necessary if baby is on a three-hour schedule.

Bottle and nipple brushes

Bottle sterilizer (should have rack so bottles can be inverted and held above water and sterilized by streaming steam. Either electric or stove top type)

Bottle warmer and vaporizer

Strainer

Funnel if using small-necked bottle

Measuring cup (If bottle is correctly marked, it can be used for measuring)

Spoon and knife or spatula to measure a level spoonful correctly

Mixing pan or pitcher

Sleeping Essentials

Crib or bassinet

Moisture-proof mattress protector

Firm mattress

Crib blankets (cotton 1 or 2; wool 1 or 2)

Receiving blankets (cotton 4 to 6)

Sheets for crib—6

Moisture-proof pads (2 bed length, 4 to 6, small)

Absorbent pads (Curity or quilted 6 to 8)

Consideration for the Doctor

Practicing obstetrics is probably the most pleasant speciality in medicine. One is constantly dealing with healthy patients who have a great joy before them, and the obstetrician is able to partake in the fulfillment of this wonderful event. Only rarely is there a sorrowful termination of a healthy pregnancy which comparatively does little to detract from the satisfaction that the accoucheur receives. With these introductory remarks the indulgence and the understanding of patients in general are sought.

The general practitioner knows little rest, and the same can be said for the busy obstetrician. Often both will attend the office after a night without sleep or following a complicated or difficult case which may have been most fatiguing. Patients can show their doctors consideration in many ways, and the following ideas are presented: (1) Do not call the doctor during the night for problems that can await his office. Save routine questions for the regular prenatal visits. But whenever you have a question, you deserve an answer. Your doctor wants you to be at ease mentally as well as physically, and this will not be possible if you wonder and worry about something troubling you, or which leaves you in doubt about its seriousness. Do not hesitate to call anytime about something that you feel is important! (2) During the prenatal visits have your questions ready and organized (preferably written down) so that when you leave the office you have the feeling that all of your questions and problems have been satisfied. (3) Should you find it necessary to call your doctor and you find him not in and you leave your number, try to keep your phone open so that he can reach you when he returns your call. (4) When calling the office for an appointment only, let the secretary make a time convenient for you; it is not necessary to consult your doctor for this.

It may be a bit presumptuous to bring these ideas before you, but in conversations with my colleagues, the greatest source of provocation is what has been mentioned here. In order to establish the closest degree of doctor-patient relationship, not only must the patient be aware that her doctor has her every interest at heart, but the doctor should be given to know that his patients consider his feelings too.

Questions and Suggestions

This space is to be used for writing down questions that arise between visits to your doctor and which might be forgotten unless noted when they occur to you. It also serves as a convenient place to record your doctor's instructions and the time of your next appointment.

First Visit   Date............................   Time........................
   Questions...

....

   Suggestions...

....

Second Visit   Date............................   Time........................
   Questions...

....

   Suggestions...

....

Third Visit   Date............................   Time........................
   Questions...

....

   Suggestions...

....

Fourth Visit   Date............................   Time........................
   Questions...

....

   Suggestions...

....

Fifth Visit   Date...................................   Time...................
     Questions...

     Suggestions...

Sixth Visit   Date...................................   Time...................
     Questions...

     Suggestions...

Seventh Visit   Date...................................   Time...................
     Questions...

     Suggestions...

Eighth Visit   Date...................................   Time...................
     Questions...

     Suggestions...

Ninth Visit   Date...................................   Time...................
     Questions...

     Suggestions...

Tenth Visit   Date...................................   Time...................
     Questions...

     Suggestions...

Eleventh Visit   Date............................   Time........................

    Questions..

    Suggestions..

Twelfth Visit   Date............................   Time........................

    Questions..

    Suggestions..

Thirteenth Visit   Date............................   Time........................

    Questions..

    Suggestions..

Fourteenth Visit   Date............................   Time........................

    Questions..

    Suggestions..

Fifteenth Visit   Date............................   Time........................

    Questions..

    Suggestions..

Names for Baby

Below are over 2,000 names that may be of some assistance in naming the new arrival. However, books with a more extensive listing are available; they include a description of the meaning of the names and their derivation.

GIRLS' NAMES

Abigail	Amethyst	Astrid	Beth	Cary	Claudia
Abby	Amity	Atalanta	Betsy	Caryn	Claudine
Ada	Amorette	Atalie	Bettinna	Cassandra	Clementine
Adalia	Amy	Athalia	Betty	Cassie	Cleo
Adelaide	Anastasia	Athena	Beulah	Catalina	Clorinda
Adele	Andrea	Auberta	Bianca	Caterina	Clotilde
Adeline	Andromeda	Audrey	Billie	Catherine	Clover
Adrienne	Angela	Audris	Blanche	Cecile	Colette
Agatha	Angelina	Augusta	Blossom	Cecilia	Colleen
Agnes	Anita	Augustina	Blythe	Celena	Columbine
Ailsa	Anitra	Aurea	Bonnibel	Celeste	Comfort
Aimee	Ann	Aurelia	Bonnie	Celestine	Constance
Alanna	Anna	Austine	Brenda	Celia	Constantia
Alberta	Annabel	Avis	Brenna	Cerelia	Consuela
Alda	Annette	Azalea	Briana	Charis	Cora
Aldis	Anthia	Babette	Bridget	Charity	Coral
Alethea	Antoinette	Baptista	Brunhilde	Charlene	Coralie
Alexandra	Antonia	Barbara	Calandra	Charlotte	Corella
Alice	April	Beatrice	Calvina	Charmain	Coretta
Alicia	Arabella	Belda	Camilla	Cherry	Corinna
Alida	Araminta	Belinda	Candace	Cheryl	Cornelia
Alina	Ardath	Bella	Candida	Chloe	Crystal
Alison	Ardelle	Belle	Cara	Chloris	Cynthia
Allegra	Ardine	Benedetta	Carilla	Christabel	Cyrene
Alma	Ardis	Benedicta	Carisa	Christel	Cytherea
Almira	Ardith	Benetta	Carita	Christiane	Dacia
Althea	Areta	Benita	Carla	Christina	Dagmar
Alva	Ariadne	Berdine	Carlen	Clara	Daisy
Alvina	Ariana	Bernadette	Carlina	Clare	Dale
Alvita	Ariella	Bernardine	Carlita	Clarette	Damaris
Amabel	Arlana	Berneta	Carlotta	Claribel	Danette
Amalea	Arlene	Bernice	Carmel	Clarice	Danila
Amanda	Arleta	Bertha	Carmen	Clarinda	Danita
Amaris	Armilda	Bertilde	Carmita	Clarine	Daphne
Amaryllis	Armilla	Bertina	Carol	Clarissa	Dara
Amber	Arva	Beryl	Carola	Clarita	Daralis
Amelia	Astra	Bess	Caroline	Claudette	Daria

Darice	Dulcy	Elspeth	Felice	Gloria	Hortense
Darlene	Easter	Elva	Felicia	Gloriane	Huberta
Daryl	Echo	Elvine	Fenella	Grace	Hulda
Davina	Eda	Elvira	Fern	Gracia	Hyacinth
Dawn	Edana	Emelda	Fernanda	Grania	Ianthe
Deanna	Eden	Emeline	Fidela	Gratiana	Ida
Deborah	Edina	Emera	Fidelity	Greer	Idalia
Delcine	Edith	Emily	Fifine	Greta	Idaline
Delia	Editha	Emlyn	Fiona	Gretchen	Idelle
Delicia	Edlyn	Emma	Flavia	Griselda	Idette
Delilah	Edmonda	Emmylou	Fleur	Guinette	Idola
Della	Edna	Enid	Fleurette	Guinevere	Idona
Delora	Edra	Enrica	Flora	Gustava	Ignacia
Deloris	Edris	Erica	Florella	Gustel	Ilka
Delphine	Edwina	Erina	Florence	Gwen	Imogen
Demetria	Effie	Ermina	Floria	Gwendolyn	Ina
Denise	Eileen	Erna	Florida	Gweneth	Inez
Desiree	Elaine	Ernesta	Floris	Gwynne	Ingrid
Desma	Elata	Ernestine	Fonda	Gypsy	Ione
Desmona	Elberta	Esme	Forrest	Halette	Irene
Devona	Eldora	Esmeralda	Frances	Hally	Iris
Diane	Eldoris	Estelle	Francesca	Hannah	Irma
Dianthe	Eldrida	Esther	Francine	Haralda	Irmina
Dinah	Eleanor	Estra	Freda	Harriet	Isabel
Dione	Electra	Estrella	Fredella	Hatty	Isidora
Dionis	Elena	Ethel	Fredrika	Hazel	Isolde
Dixie	Eleonora	Ethelda	Fritzi	Heather	Iva
Docilla	Elfreda	Ethelind	Gabrielle	Hebe	Ivy
Dolly	Elida	Etta	Gail	Hedda	Jacinta
Dolores	Elise	Eudocia	Galatea	Hedwig	Jacqueline
Domela	Elissa	Eudora	Garda	Helen	Jane
Dominica	Elita	Eugenia	Garland	Helene	Janella
Donalda	Eliza	Eulalia	Garnet	Heloise	Janet
Donata	Elizabeth	Eunice	Gay	Helga	Janice
Donella	Ella	Eva	Geneva	Helsa	Jaquenette
Donica	Elladine	Evangeline	Genevieve	Henrietta	Jarita
Donna	Ellamay	Evania	Georgette	Henrika	Jasmine
Dora	Ellen	Evanthe	Georgia	Hera	Jean
Doralia	Ellette	Eve	Georgina	Hermandine	Jeanne
Doralis	Ellice	Eveleen	Geralda	Hermia	Jeannette
Dorcas	Elma	Evelyn	Geraldine	Hermione	Jemima
Dorette	Elmina	Fabrienne	Germaine	Hesper	Jennifer
Doria	Elna	Faith	Gertrude	Hester	Jenny
Dorice	Elnora	Fanchon	Gilberte	Hetty	Jessica
Doris	Elodie	Fania	Gilda	Hilda	Jewel
Dorita	Eloine	Fanny	Gizella	Hildegard	Jill
Dorlisa	Eloise	Fay	Gladys	Hollis	Joan
Dorothea	Elora	Fayette	Glenda	Holly	Jobyna
Dorothy	Elsa	Fedora	Glenna	Honora	Jocelyn
Dulcia	Elsie	Felda	Glennis	Hope	Johanna

Josephine	Letitia	Mabel	Maude	Nadine	Oriel
Joy	Letty	Madel	Maura	Nan	Orlantha
Joyce	Lexine	Madeleine	Maurella	Nana	Orlena
Juanita	Liane	Madge	Maureen	Nancy	Orva
Judith	Libby	Madra	Maurita	Nanelle	Osa
Judy	Lila	Mae	Mavia	Nanette	Ouida
Julia	Lilith	Magdalen	Mavis	Nanine	Pamela
Juliana	Lillian	Maggie	Mavra	Naomi	Pandora
Julienne	Lily	Magnolia	Maxine	Nara	Pansy
Juliet	Lilybell	Maisie	May	Narda	Parthenia
Julita	Linda	Malina	Maya	Natala	Patience
June	Lisa	Malva	Maybelle	Natalie	Patricia
Juno	Lisabetta	Manda	Mayda	Natasha	Paula
Justine	Lise	Manette	Medora	Nathania	Paulette
Kara	Lisette	Manon	Meg	Neala	Pauline
Karen	Livia	Manuela	Megan	Nedda	Paulita
Karla	Lois	Mara	Melanie	Nelda	Peace
Kasia	Lola	Maraline	Melantha	Nelia	Pearl
Kate	Lolita	Marcella	Melinda	Nell	Peggy
Katherine	Lona	Marcelline	Melissa	Nella	Penelope
Kathleen	Lore	Marcia	Melita	Nellis	Peony
Katrina	Lorelei	Marea	Melva	Nerine	Pepita
Kay	Lorelle	Marelda	Melvina	Nerissa	Persis
Kelda	Lorena	Marella	Mercedes	Nerita	Petrina
Kirstie	Loretta	Maretta	Mercia	Nessa	Philana
Koren	Lorinda	Margaret	Mercy	Netty	Philippa
Lalita	Loris	Margarita	Merle	Neysa	Phillida
Lara	Lorita	Margot	Merry	Nicolette	Philomela
Larissa	Lorna	Marguerite	Meryl	Nina	Philomena
Latona	Lorraine	Maria	Meta	Ninette	Phoebe
Laura	Lotta	Marian	Mignon	Ninon	Phyllis
Laurel	Lotus	Marianne	Mildred	Noel	Pierrette
Laurella	Louise	Maribel	Milicent	Nola	Pippa
Laurene	Lucia	Marice	Milly	Nolita	Polly
Lauretta	Luciana	Marie	Mimi	Nona	Pollyanna
Laverne	Lucie	Mariel	Minerva	Nora	Pomona
Lavinia	Lucilla	Marietta	Minna	Norine	Poppy
Leah	Lucille	Marigold	Minnie	Norma	Portia
Leila	Lucina	Marilyn	Mirabelle	Nydia	Primrose
Lelah	Lucinda	Marina	Miranda	Octavia	Priscilla
Lena	Lucrece	Marjorie	Miriam	Ola	Prudence
Lenore	Lucretia	Marla	Molly	Olethea	Prunella
Leola	Lucy	Marlene	Mona	Olga	Queena
Leona	Luella	Marta	Monica	Olive	Quenby
Leonora	Lulito	Martella	Muriel	Olivia	Quentina
Leontine	Lulu	Martha	Myra	Olympia	Rachel
Leora	Lydia	Martina	Myrilla	Opal	Rae
Leslie	Lynette	Mary	Myrna	Ophelia	Ramona
Leta	Lynn	Maryann	Myrtle	Ora	Rana
Lethia	Lyris	Matilda	Nada	Oribel	Raphaela

Reba	Rosetta	Sira	Thadine	Ursula	Vivian
Rebbecca	Rosina	Sigrid	Thais	Vaile	Vivienne
Regina	Rowena	Silva	Thalia	Val	Wanda
Rena	Roxane	Silver	Thea	Valda	Wendelin
Renata	Rubetta	Simone	Theda	Valeda	Wendy
Renee	Ruby	Sirena	Thelma	Valencia	Wenona
Renita	Ruth	Solita	Theodora	Valentina	Wilda
Rhea	Sabine	Sonia	Theodosia	Valerie	Wilfreda
Rhoda	Sabrina	Sophia	Theola	Valora	Wilhelmina
Ricarda	Sadie	Stacy	Thera	Vanessa	Willa
Rita	Sadira	Starr	Theresa	Vania	Willabel
Roberta	Sally	Stella	Thisbe	Vara	Willow
Robina	Salome	Stephanie	Thyra	Veda	Wilma
Robinette	Samara	Sue	Tina	Vedette	Winifred
Rochelle	Samuela	Susan	Tobey	Vedis	Wynne
Roderica	Sandra	Susanna	Tonia	Velda	Yetta
Rolanda	Sapphira	Susanne	Trella	Veleda	Yolanda
Romola	Sarah	Suzette	Trilby	Vera	Yseult
Ronalda	Sarita	Sydney	Trina	Verda	Yvette
Rosa	Selena	Sylvana	Trinette	Verna	Yvonne
Rosabel	Seleta	Sylvia	Trista	Vernita	Zandra
Rosalie	Selma	Tabitha	Trude	Veronica	Zaneta
Rosalind	Senalda	Tallula	Trudel	Victoria	Zelda
Rosalyn	Serena	Tamara	Udele	Victorine	Zenia
Rosamond	Serilda	Tara	Ula	Vida	Zita
Rosanna	Sharon	Teresa	Ulrica	Vidette	Zoe
Rose	Sheila	Teresina	Una	Viola	Zora
Rosel	Shirley	Tertia	Urania	Violet	Zorana
Rosemarie	Sibyl	Tess	Ursa	Virginia	
Rosemary	Sidonia	Tessa	Ursel	Vita	

BOYS' NAMES

Aaron	Adin	Alden	Alton	Anson	Asher
Abbot	Adley	Aldis	Alvar	Anthony	Ashford
Abel	Adolph	Aldrich	Alvin	Anton	Ashley
Abelard	Adrian	Aldwin	Alvis	Archer	Ashton
Abner	Ahern	Alexander	Alwin	Archibald	Athmore
Abraham	Aiken	Alford	Ambrose	Arden	Atwater
Abram	Ainsley	Alfred	Amery	Arlen	Atwell
Absalom	Ainsworth	Alger	Amiel	Arley	Atwood
Ackley	Alair	Algernon	Amos	Armand	Aubrey
Adair	Alan	Alison	Anatol	Armin	August
Adalard	Alaric	Allen	Anders	Armstrong	Augustus
Adam	Alban	Alonzo	Anderson	Arnold	Austin
Adams	Albern	Alphonse	Andrew	Arthur	Averill
Adamson	Albert	Alroy	Angelo	Arvin	Avery
Addis	Albion	Alson	Angus	Asa	Axel
Addison	Alcott	Alston	Anselm	Ashby	Aylmer

Aylsworth	Bradley	Chapman	Dallas	Edan	Fabian
Bailey	Bradwell	Chappell	Dalton	Edgar	Fabron
Bainbridge	Brandon	Charles	Damon	Edmund	Fairfax
Baird	Brant	Cheney	Dana	Edsel	Farley
Baldwin	Brent	Chester	Daniel	Edson	Farrel
Bancroft	Brett	Christian	Darcy	Edward	Felix
Barclay	Brewster	Christopher	Darnell	Edwin	Fenton
Barlow	Brian	Clarence	Darrell	Egan	Ferdinand
Barnaby	Brice	Clark	Darrick	Egbert	Fergus
Barney	Brigham	Claude	Darton	Egerton	Fernald
Barrett	Brock	Clay	David	Elbert	Ferris
Barron	Broderick	Clayborn	Davin	Elden	Fitzgerald
Barry	Bromley	Clayton	Davis	Eli	Fitzpatrick
Bartholomew	Bronson	Clement	Dean	Elias	Flavian
Bartlett	Brooks	Clifford	Dearborn	Elihu	Fletcher
Bartley	Bruce	Clifton	Delmar	Elijah	Florian
Barton	Bruno	Clinton	Delwin	Eliot	Floyd
Basil	Bryant	Clive	Dempster	Elisha	Forbes
Baxter	Burgess	Clyde	Dennis	Ellery	Forrest
Bayard	Burke	Colby	Denton	Ellis	Foster
Benedict	Burleigh	Colin	Dermot	Ellison	Fowler
Benjamin	Byron	Collis	Derrick	Elmer	Francis
Bennett	Caesar	Colman	Derwin	Elroy	Frank
Bentley	Caleb	Colton	Desmond	Elton	Franklin
Benton	Calvert	Condon	Devin	Elwin	Fred
Berkeley	Calvin	Conrad	Dexter	Ely	Frederick
Bernard	Cameron	Conroy	Dickson	Emanuel	Freedland
Bert	Campbell	Conway	Dillon	Emerson	Fritz
Berton	Carew	Corbin	Dinsmore	Emery	Freeman
Bertram	Carey	Corey	Dion	Emil	Gabriel
Berwin	Carl	Cornelius	Dirk	Emmet	Gail
Bevan	Carlisle	Corwin	Dominic	Enoch	Galvin
Beverley	Carlton	Courtland	Don	Enos	Gardner
Bevis	Carney	Courtney	Donald	Ephraim	Garland
Blaine	Carroll	Craig	Dorian	Eric	Garner
Blair	Carson	Crandall	Douglas	Ernald	Garrett
Blake	Carter	Crawford	Doyle	Ernest	Garrick
Blandon	Carvel	Creighton	Drew	Errol	Garvin
Bolton	Carver	Cromwell	Driscoll	Erskine	Gary
Booth	Cary	Crosby	Dudley	Erwin	Gaston
Borden	Casey	Cullen	Duke	Esmond	Geoffrey
Boris	Casimir	Culver	Duncan	Ethan	George
Bowden	Cecil	Curt	Durant	Ethelbert	Gerald
Bowen	Cedric	Curtis	Durward	Eugene	Gerard
Boyce	Chadburn	Cuthbert	Durwin	Eustace	Gifford
Boyd	Chadwick	Cutler	Dwight	Evan	Gilbert
Boyden	Chalmer	Cuyler	Earl	Everett	Giles
Boynton	Chandler	Cyril	Eaton	Evers	Gilford
Braden	Channing	Cyrus	Eben	Ezekiel	Gilfred
Bradford	Chapin	Dale	Ebenezer	Ezra	Gilmer

Gilmore	Herman	Jock	Lane	Maitland	Morton
Gladwin	Heyward	Joel	Lang	Malcolm	Moses
Glen	Hilary	John	Langley	Mallory	Munro
Glendon	Hilton	Johnston	Lars	Malvin	Murdock
Goddard	Hilliard	Jonas	Latham	Mandel	Murray
Godfrey	Hiram	Jonathan	Lathrop	Manton	Myron
Godwin	Hobart	Jordan	Latimer	Manuelle	Nathan
Gordon	Holbrook	Joseph	Lawrence	Manvel	Nathaniel
Graham	Holden	Joshua	Lawton	Marcel	Neal
Grant	Hollis	Josiah	Leander	Marcus	Nehemiah
Grantland	Holman	Jules	Lee	Marion	Nelson
Grayson	Holmes	Julian	Leigh	Marius	Nestor
Gregory	Homer	Julius	Leighton	Mark	Neville
Griffith	Horace	Justin	Leith	Marland	Nevin
Grover	Howard	Karl	Leland	Marlow	Newton
Gustavus	Howland	Karsten	Leo	Marsden	Nicholas
Guthrie	Hubert	Keane	Leon	Marshall	Nigel
Guy	Hugh	Keegan	Leonard	Marston	Niles
Hadley	Hugo	Keith	Leopold	Martin	Noah
Haines	Humphrey	Kelby	Leroy	Marvin	Noel
Hal	Hunt	Kelsey	Leslie	Mason	Nolan
Halbert	Huntley	Kelvin	Lester	Mathias	Norbert
Hale	Hyman	Kendall	Levi	Matthew	Norman
Halford	Ian	Kenley	Lew	Maurice	Norris
Hall	Ichabod	Kenneth	Lincoln	Max	Norton
Hallam	Ignace	Kent	Lindsay	Maxwell	Norval
Halsey	Ingram	Kenton	Lionel	Maynard	Norvin
Hamilton	Ira	Kenway	Livingston	Mead	Oakes
Hamlin	Irvin	Kenyon	Llewellyn	Melville	Oakley
Hampton	Irving	Kermit	Lloyd	Melvin	Odell
Hanford	Irwin	Kerry	Lockwood	Mercer	Ogden
Hanley	Isaac	Kerwin	Logan	Meredith	Olaf
Hans	Isaiah	Kester	Lombard	Merrick	Olin
Hansel	Isidore	Kevin	Loren	Merrill	Oliver
Harcourt	Israel	Kilby	Lorimer	Merton	Olney
Hardy	Ivan	Kim	Lorin	Merwin	Orin
Harlan	Ivar	Kimball	Loring	Meyer	Orlando
Harley	Jack	Kingdom	Louis	Michael	Ormond
Harold	Jacob	Kingsley	Lowell	Milburn	Orson
Harris	James	Kingston	Lucius	Miles	Orton
Harry	Jarvis	Kirby	Ludlow	Miller	Orville
Hartley	Jason	Kirk	Luke	Milton	Orvin
Hartwell	Jasper	Konrad	Luther	Mitchell	Osborn
Harvey	Jay	Kurt	Lydell	Montague	Oscar
Hayden	Jed	Laird	Lyle	Moreland	Osgood
Hayes	Jeffrey	Lambert	Lyman	Morgan	Osmond
Heath	Jeremy	Lamont	Lynn	Morley	Oswald
Hector	Jerome	Landers	Macnair	Morrell	Otis
Henry	Jerrold	Landon	Madison	Morris	Otto
Herbert	Jesse	Landry	Magnus	Mortimer	Ovid

Owen	Raphael	Sawyer	Stewart	Ulric	Welford
Page	Ray	Schuyler	Stillman	Ulysses	Wellington
Paine	Rayburn	Scott	Stilwell	Upton	Wells
Palmer	Raymond	Seabrook	Stoddard	Uriah	Wendell
Park	Redmund	Searle	Sumner	Vail	Wesley
Parker	Regan	Sebastian	Sutton	Val	Weston
Patrick	Reginald	Selby	Sylvester	Valdis	Whitby
Paul	Reid	Seldon	Talbot	Vance	Whitelaw
Paxton	Rendell	Selwyn	Taylor	Vandyke	Whitford
Pearson	Reuben	Serge	Tearle	Van Ness	Whitney
Pedro	Rex	Seth	Tedmund	Varick	Wilbur
Pembroke	Rexford	Seton	Terence	Varney	Wildon
Penrod	Reynold	Seward	Terrill	Vaughn	Wilford
Percival	Richard	Sewell	Terris	Verne	Wilfred
Percy	Richmond	Seymour	Thaddeus	Vernon	Will
Perrin	Ripley	Shaw	Thatcher	Victor	Willard
Perry	Robert	Shawn	Thaxter	Vincent	William
Peter	Robin	Shelby	Thayer	Vinson	Willis
Phelan	Roderick	Sheldon	Theobald	Virgil	Wilmer
Phelps	Rodman	Shelley	Theodore	Vivien	Wilmot
Philander	Rodney	Shepherd	Theodoric	Wade	Wilson
Philbert	Roger	Shepley	Thomas	Wadsworth	Wilton
Philip	Roland	Sheridan	Thornton	Walbridge	Winchell
Phineas	Rolfe	Sherlock	Thorpe	Walcott	Windsor
Pierce	**Rollin**	Sherman	Thurlow	Waldemar	Winfield
Pierpont	Rollo	Sherwin	Thurston	Walden	Winfred
Pierre	Romney	Sherwood	Tilden	Waldo	Winslow
Pierson	Ronald	Sidney	Tilford	Waldon	Winston
Powell	Roscoe	Siegfried	Timothy	Waldron	Winthrop
Prentice	Ross	Sigmund	Titus	Walford	Wolcott
Prescott	Roy	Silas	Tobias	Walker	Wolfe
Preston	Royce	Simon	Tobin	Walt	Wolfram
Prince	Royd	Simpson	Tolman	Wallace	Woodley
Prior	Rudolph	Sinclair	Tom	Walter	Woodman
Proctor	Rufus	Sloan	Tony	Walton	Woodrow
Prosper	Rupert	Sol	Torbert	Ward	Woodward
Putnam	Russell	Solomon	Torrance	Ware	Worden
Quentin	Rutherford	Spencer	Torrey	Warfield	Worthington
Quincy	Sabin	Sprague	Townsend	Warford	Wright
Quinn	Salisbury	Stacy	Tracy	Waring	Wyatt
Radburn	**Sam**	Stafford	Trahern	Warner	Wylie
Radcliffe	Sampson	Standish	Travis	Warren	Wyman
Radford	Samuel	Stanfield	Trent	Warrick	Wyndham
Radley	Sanborn	Stanford	Trevor	Warton	Xavier
Raleigh	Sanders	**Stanley**	Tristan	Washington	Yardley
Ralph	Sandon	Stanton	Truman	Watson	Yates
Ralston	Sandor	Stanway	Tucker	Wayland	York
Ramon	Sanford	Stanwood	Tully	Wayne	Zachary
Ramsey	Sargent	Stephan	Turner	Webb	Zane
Randall	Saul	Sterling	Tyler	Webster	
Randolph	Saville	Steven	Tyson	Weldon	

Birthstones

These precious stones are considered appropriate to, or symbolizing the influences due to, the month or the day of one's birth.

January	garnet	Sunday	topaz and diamond
February	amethyst	Monday	pearl and crystal
March	jasper or bloodstone	Tuesday	ruby and emerald
April	diamond or sapphire	Wednesday	amethyst and loadstone
May	emerald	Thursday	sapphire and carnelian
June	agate	Friday	emerald and cat's-eye
July	turquoise	Saturday	turquoise and diamond
August	carnelian		
September	chrysolite		
October	beryl		
November	topaz		
December	ruby		

Glossary

abnormal. Irregular, deviating from the natural or standard type.

abortion. Interruption of pregnancy before the fetus is capable of independent existence, i.e., before it is developed 26 weeks.

afterbirth. The round flat vascular organ which nourishes the child in the uterus—the placenta.

amenorrhea. Absence of menstruation.

amnesia. Loss of memory.

amnion. Inner layer of the sac in which the fetus lies.

amniotic fluid. The fluid in which the fetus is suspended, i.e., the fluid of the bag of waters.

analgesic. An agent which abolishes the sense of pain, but does not necessarily cause loss of consciousness.

anatomy. The science of the structure of the body and the relation of its parts.

anemia. A deficiency of some of the constituents of the blood.

anesthetic. An agent which produces loss of sensibility to pain.

antepartum. Before delivery.

antiseptic. An agent which destroys bacteria.

areola. The darkish area around the nipple.

Aschheim-Zondek test. A laboratory test for pregnancy in which the patient's blood or urine is in-

jected into a mouse. There are closely related tests in which a rabbit or other animal may be used.

asepsis. The exclusion of disease-producing bacteria.

asphyxia. A condition caused by failure of respiration, due to lack of oxygen and carbon dioxide.

bacteria. Microscopic one-celled organisms.

birth canal. The passage through which the child is born.

breech. The buttocks.

calorie. The unit ordinarily employed by nutritionists to measure energy-producing value of food.

cardiac. Pertaining to the heart.

cardiovascular. Pertaining to the heart and blood vessels.

catheterize. To empty the bladder by means of a tubelike instrument which is introduced into the passage through which the urine normally leaves the bladder.

cautery. The application of a caustic substance or of a hot iron.

cesarean section. Removal of the child by incision through the walls of the abdomen and uterus when delivery through the normal passage is not advisable.

chemotherapy. The treatment or prevention of disease by the use of specific chemical drugs.

chorionic membrane. The outermost of the two membranes which surround the embryo.

chromosomes. Rodlike bodies in the nucleus of the cell. They are composed of innumerable genes which in the sperm and ova are the carriers of hereditary qualities.

climacteric. The time of the ending of menstruation; the phase of the menopause.

clitoris. A pea-sized erectile organ of sexual significance at the top of the vulva.

coitus. Sexual intercourse.

colostrum. The fluid secreted by the breast just before or after the birth of the baby.

conception. The fertilization of the ovum.

contagious. Transmitted from one person to another.

contraception. Prevention of pregnancy.

contractions. Shortening of muscle fibers of the uterus to press upon its contents. In obstetrics it means a labor pain.

copulation. Sexual congress or coitus.

corpus luteum. A yellow mass in the ovary formed by a graafian follicle which has matured and discharged its ovum.

curettage. A scraping of the womb to remove tissue or blood clots.

diagnosis. Determination of either normal or abnormal states of the body.

diaphragm. The muscular partition between the chest and abdomen. Also, a contraceptive device.

disproportion. The condition where the baby is relatively larger than the passages of the mother.

duct. A tube which conveys the secretion from a gland.

dysmenorrhea. Painful menstruation.

dyspnea. Difficult or labored breathing.

eclampsia. A sudden attack of convulsions or coma, or both, usually occurring during the last three months of pregnancy, and associated with high blood pressure, edema, and albumin in the urine.

ectopic. Out of the normal place.

edema. Swelling due to accumulation of fluid in the tissues of the body.

embryo. The fetus in its earlier stages of development, especially before the end of the third month.

embryology. The science which treats of the development of the embryo.

endocrine. Applied to organs whose function is to secrete hormones into the blood.

epigastrium. The upper middle portion of the abdomen, over or in front of the stomach.

erythroblastosis. A blood disease of the unborn fetus, or of the newborn baby due to mother-child blood incompatibility on a parental basis.

excretion. Waste substance thrown off from the body.

extra-uterine pregnancy. Pregnancy developing outside the uterine cavity; an ectopic pregnancy.

extremities. The legs and arms.

fertile. Capable of reproduction.

fetus. The fully formed child after the third month of pregnancy until birth.

fontanelle. Any one of the soft spots of the head of a young infant.

gamete. A sexual cell.

generative organs. Pertaining to the reproductive organs.

gestation. Pregnancy.

gland. An organ which separates material from the blood and manufactures a secretion. Most glands discharge their secretions through a duct, but the glands of internal secretion are ductless (the endocrine glands).

gonorrhea. Venereal infection due to the gonococcus.

graafian follicle. Any one of the small vesicular sacs imbedded in the cortex of the ovary, each of which contains an ovum.

gynecology. The study of diseases peculiar to women.

hormone. A chemical substance produced in an endocrine gland and carried by the blood stream to other parts of the body where it excites a functional activity.

hygiene. The science or system of principles devoted to the preservation of health and the prevention of disease.

implantation. The embedding of the fertilized ovum in the womb for purposes of growth and development.

impregnation. The fertilization of an egg by a sperm. The act of rendering pregnant.

infection. Invasion of the body by harmful bacteria.

intestines. The bowels; the long membranous tube extending from the stomach to the rectum.

involution. Return of the pelvic organs to their normal condition after childbirth.

jaundice. Yellowness of the skin, eyes and secretions due to the presence of bile pigments in the blood.

lactation. Formation and secretion of milk.

latent. Concealed.

leukorrhea. A whitish, viscid discharge from the vagina.

ligate. To tie off with a ligature.

lobes. Subdivisions or portions of the breast.

lochia. A discharge present for about two weeks after the birth of the child.

lunar month. A month of 28 days.

mammary. Relating to the breast.

mature. Ripe or fully developed.

meconium. The fecal matter discharged by the newborn, a dark green substance.

menopause. The period when menstruation normally ceases; the change of life.

menstruation. The monthly bleeding.

metabolism. The building up and breaking down of body tissues.

metamorphosis. Change of shape or structure.

miscarriage. The same as abortion.

Montgomery's tubercles. Sebaceous glands of the mammary areola.

mucous membrane. The membrane which lines canals and cavities, which communicate with external air; an example is the vagina.

multipara. A woman who has borne more than one child.

narcotics. Drugs which produce sleep.

navel. The place in the abdomen where the cord was attached which connected the baby with the mother.

neurotic. A nervous person in whom emotions predominate over reason.

obese. Excessively fat.

obstetrics. The art and science which has for its field human reproduction.

ovary. The female sex gland in which the ova lie and where hormones are produced.

ovulation. The formation and discharge of an unimpregnated ovum from the graafian follicle of the ovary.

ovum. An egg; the female reproductive cell of the ovary.

palpate. To examine by the hand.

pathology. The branch of medicine which deals with the altered structure and activity of diseased organs.

pediatrician. A specialist in the treatment of children's diseases.

pelvic floor. The sling of muscles and other tissue which support the bottom of the pelvic basin.

pelvis. The bony passages through which the baby must pass in a delivery by way of the vagina.

perineum. The area between the outlet of the vagina and the rectum; an integral part of the pelvic floor.

physiologic. Pertaining to the functions of the body and organs.

pigmentation. The coloration or discoloration of the skin by a pigment.

pituitary. The "master" gland of the body; the hypophysis.

placenta. The round, flat vascular organ within the uterus which establishes communication between the mother and child by means of the umbilical cord; the afterbirth.

prenatal. Occurring during pregnancy, i.e., before the birth.

primigravida. A woman pregnant for the first time.

primipara. A woman who has given birth to only one child.

progesterone. The hormone from the corpus luteum.

prophylactic. Tending to ward off disease; preventative.

psychosomatics. The study of the inter-relationship of mind and body.

puberty. The age at which the reproductive organs become functional.

puerperal fever. Infection following childbirth.

puerperium. The interval following the birth of the child during which the mother's body returns to the normal, healthy, nonpregnant state.

purulent. Consisting of or containing pus.

quickening. The first recognizable movements of the fetus sensed by the mother.

Rh factor. A variable factor in the blood important in its relationship to erythroblastosis.

semen. The thick, whitish, liquid secretion produced by the male during intercourse.

spermatozoon. The motile generative element of the semen which impregnates the ovum.

spontaneous. Occurring naturally, without aid.

sterility. Inability to become pregnant.

striae. Lines or streaks seen upon the abdomen, breasts and buttocks of pregnant women.

symptom. Any evidence of a disease or of a patient's condition. *Subjective.* One that is perceptible to the patient only. *Objective.* One that is obvious to an observer.

syphilis. A venereal infection of the blood, due to the spirochete Treponema pallida.

term. The time of expected delivery.

therapeutic. Concerned with the treatment of disease.

tubes. The oviducts.

toxemia. A condition occurring toward the end of pregnancy, attended by high blood pressure, marked edema, and albumin in the urine and certain symptoms.

trimester. The pregnancy is divided into three periods of three months each; each period is known as a trimester.

umbilical cord. The navel string which carries the blood vessels passing between the placenta and the child's navel.

uterus. The womb; a muscular, hollow organ which receives, retains, nourishes and finally expels the baby.

vagina. The canal through which the child passes from the uterus into the world.

vernix. The fatty substance deposited over the skin of the newly born infant.

viable. Capable of living outside of the uterus.

villi. The microscopic, finger-like processes which hang from one of the surfaces of the placenta and are surrounded by the mother's blood.

vitamins. Accessory food substances essential for growth and health, the lack of which causes certain deficiency diseases like rickets and scurvy.

vulva. The external female generative organs.

Wassermann. A blood test for syphilis.

zygote. The cell resulting from the fusion of two gametes.

Index